The HUNGER HERO DIET

Fast and easy recipe series #1

Cooking with
FISH

Kathryn M. James

Copyright © 2022 by Kathryn M James

All Rights Reserved.

No part of this book may be used or reproduced by any means, graphic, electronic, or mechanical, including photocopying, recording, taping, or by any information storage retrieval system without the written permission of the copyright owner, except in the case of brief quotations embodied in critical articles and reviews.

The Working Alliance, Gold Coast, Australia
ISBN 978-0-6455255-3-3

kmjameswriter.com

This edition may contain product information specific to the supermarket shopping experience in Australasia.

Disclaimer

Neither the author nor the publisher can be held liable to any person or entity with respect to any loss or damage caused, or alleged to be caused, directly or indirectly, by the information contained in this work or associated media. As any scientist will affirm, results may vary, so no guarantee is given or implied with regard to information supplied. It is general information only.

It is not the intent of the author to diagnose or prescribe. The intent is only to offer health information to help you cooperate with your medical professionals in your mutual quest for health. In the event you use this information without their approval, you are prescribing for yourself, which is your right, but the publisher and author assume no responsibility. While every precaution has been taken to ensure the information presented herein is accurate, there are many factors beyond the control of the author.

Before starting any diet, you should speak to your doctor. Do not rely on information in this book as an alternative to medical advice. If you have any specific questions about any medical matter, consult your medical practitioner.

All trademarks or brand names mentioned by the author, in this book or elsewhere, remain unreservedly the property of their respective owners, and no claim is made to them, and no endorsement by them is implied or claimed.

Table of Contents

INTRODUCTION..........10
- How to cook CRISPY SKIN fish..........13
- How to PAN-FRY tuna steaks..........14
- How to PAN-FRY thin fish fillets..........15
- How to STEAM thin fish fillets..........16
- How to BRAISE thick fish fillets..........17
- How to make rice paper rolls..........18
- How to prepare rice noodles..........21
- How to add flavour..........24
- How to eat the rainbow..........26

TUNA STEAKS..........28
1. Tuna rolls, fennel, jalapenos..........29
2. Tuna rolls, chili, cranberry sauce..........30
3. Tuna rolls, fresh ginger, basil..........31
4. Tuna rolls, avo, sambal oelek..........32
5. Tuna rolls, avo, lemon juice..........33
6. Tuna rolls, tahini, black olives..........34
7. Tuna rolls, avo, jalapenos..........35
8. Tuna rolls, medium rare, pineapple..........36
9. Tuna rolls, nori, Asian salad..........37
10. Tuna rolls, jalapenos, coleslaw..........38
11. Rare tuna rolls, coleslaw, ginger..........39

12.	Rare tuna rolls, sesame, balsamic	40
13.	Balsamic salad rolls, with tuna	41
14.	Coleslaw rolls, spicy tuna	42
15.	Coleslaw rolls, cranberry, tuna	43
16.	Asian salad rolls, crispy tuna	44
17.	Coleslaw rolls, avo, chili tuna	45
18.	Coleslaw rolls, avo, crispy tuna	46
19.	Coleslaw rolls, tuna, asparagus	47
20.	Tuna rolls, Asian greens, herbs	48
21.	Tuna rolls, cottage cheese, silverbeet	49
22.	Sesame tuna rolls, asparagus, bok choy	50
23.	Tuna rolls, broccolini, fennel	51
24.	Green chili tuna rolls, nori, broccolini	52
25.	Chili tuna rolls, Caesar dressing	53
26.	Chili tuna rolls, asparagus, spicy dressing	54
27.	Green chili tuna rolls, pineapple	55
28.	Chili tuna rolls, fried greens	56
29.	Guacamole salad rolls, chili tuna	57
30.	Pan-fried tuna, tomato, pepita, salad	58
31.	Pan-fried tuna, asparagus, salad bowl	59
32.	Pan-fried tuna, silverbeet, asparagus	60
33.	Pan-fried tuna bowl, greens, lemon	61
34.	Pan-fried tuna bowl, broccoli	62
35.	Garlic tuna bowl, Pad Thai stir-fry	63

36. Pan-fried tuna bowl, tomato, olives...................64
37. Pan-fried tuna bowl, sweet potato, veg..............65
38. Pan-fried tuna bowl, veg, avocado.....................66
39. Pan-fried tuna, mushrooms, greens..................67
40. Pan-fried tuna, asparagus, noodle salad............68
41. Pan-fried tuna, balsamic, noodle salad..............69
42. Pan-fried tuna, silverbeet, noodle salad.............70
43. Pan-fried tuna, chilled noodle salad..................71
44. Pan-fried tuna, pineapple, noodle salad.............72
45. Pan-fried tuna, stir-fried veg, noodles................73
46. Pan-fried tuna, hoisin veg, flat noodles..............74
47. Braised tuna, miso, noodles................................75
48. Braised tuna Tom Yum, chili, noodles...............76
49. Braised tuna, yellow curry noodle soup.............77
50. Poached Malaysian tuna, flat noodles................78
51. Poached miso tuna soup, flat noodles................79
52. Instant pho, tuna, bok choy, flat noodles...........80

NEW ZEALAND HOKI..81

53. Hoki rolls, avo, jalapenos....................................82
54. Hoki rolls, alfalfa, cos lettuce..............................83
55. Hoki rolls, capers, avo...84
56. Hoki rolls, capers, sambal oelek.........................85
57. Hoki rolls, garlic, chili...86
58. Hoki rolls, beetroot, cottage cheese...................87

59. Hoki rolls, avo, onion, lime................................88
60. Hoki rolls, avo, yoghurt....................................89
61. Hoki rolls, avo, coleslaw..................................90
62. Hoki rolls, chili, crispy onion sprinkles............91
63. Hoki rolls, nori, cos lettuce............................92
64. Hoki rolls, garlic, chili, nori............................93
65. Hoki rolls, onion, nori, herbs........................94
66. Hoki rolls, nori, wasabi, kale........................95
67. Hoki rolls, chili, Mizuna salad......................96
68. Hoki rolls, fried red capsicum, nori..............97
69. Hoki rolls, fried onion, cottage cheese........98
70. Hoki rolls, fried onion, bok choy, chili.........99
71. Hoki rolls, broccolini, avo...........................100
72. Hoki rolls, pineapple, broccolini.................101
73. Hoki rolls, fried onion, asparagus..............102
74. Pan-fried Hoki, balsamic salad..................103
75. Steamed Hoki, prawns, Tom Yum..............104
76. Steamed Hoki, curry, greens, avo..............105
77. Steamed Hoki, Tom Yum, veg....................106
78. Steamed Hoki, Tamarind, Tom Yum...........107
79. Steamed Hoki, peas, Tom Yum..................108
80. Hoki egg bacon pea scramble...................109
81. Braised Hoki, prawn, Tom Yum..................110
82. Braised Hoki Tom Yum, plum sauce..........111

83. Hoki, onion, lemongrass noodle salad..............112
84. Hoki, garlic, fennel, avo, noodle bowl..............113
85. Hoki, Asian greens, Hoisin, noodle..............114
86. Hoki, mushroom, veg noodles..............115
87. Hoki Tom Yum, chili, noodle soup..............116
88. Hoki Tom Yum, Hoisin noodle soup..............117

WHITING..............118

89. Whiting rolls, passata curry..............119
90. Whiting rolls, chili, green beans..............120
91. Pan-fried whiting, chili, soy, sesame bowl..............121
92. Whiting, wombok, Tom Yum soup..............122
93. Whiting, tomato, Tom Yum noodles..............123
94. Whiting, tomato, peas, noodle soup..............124

BARRAMUNDI..............125

95. Barra rolls, avo, sambal oelek..............126
96. Barra rolls, Asian greens, avo..............127
97. Avo rolls, spicy fried barra, greens..............128
98. Pan-fried barra, garlic, capsicum, avo..............129
99. Pan-fried barra, capers, beetroot bowl..............130
100. Braised wild barramundi, veg bowl..............131
101. Braised barra, passata, veg bowl..............132
102. Braised barra, bok choy, soup bowl..............133
103. Barramundi PHO soup..............134
104. Crispy skin barra, dill, rolls..............135

105.	Crispy skin barra, ginger, rolls	136
106.	Crispy skin barra, salad bowl	137
107.	Pan-fried barra, tomato, noodle bowl	138

RED EMPEROR..139

108.	Crispy skin Red Emperor rolls	140

NORWEGIAN TROUT..141

109.	Crispy skin trout, nori, rolls	142
110.	Crispy skin trout, garlic, fried veg, rolls	144
111.	Smoked ocean trout rolls	146

TASMANIAN SALMON..147

112.	Crispy skin salmon, tartare sauce, rolls	148
113.	Pan-fried salmon cutlet, vegetables	149
114.	Smoked salmon pepper rolls	150
	About the author	151
	Titles in the HUNGER HERO series	152

INTRODUCTION

This recipe series showcases low-calorie and highly nutritious ways to prepare simple foods, following the principles of the ground-breaking HUNGER HERO DIET©.

Each of these special editions can be used as a standalone set of recipes, or as a companion to the original 300-page book:

The HUNGER HERO DIET©: How to Lose Weight and Break the Depression Cycle – Without Exercise, Drugs, or Surgery.

FISH is highly nutritious and low in calories – a perfect combination if you want to lose weight, lower blood pressure, lower triglycerides, reduce inflammation, increase HDL cholesterol, or improve insulin/glucose regulation. And the omega-3s help control appetite too (by improving *leptin* sensitivity) (Abete *et al.*, 2010). But too few people know how to prepare it, beyond deep-frying at a fish-n-chip shop – which is undeniably delicious on rare occasions, but not healthy.

In this instalment, we focus is on HOW TO COOK FISH that is highly nutritious, and fast and easy to prepare, using FRESH and FROZEN fillets we can buy in major Australian supermarkets. Most recipes are Vietnamese-inspired, focussing on flavour and texture, making the most of what you have in your fridge, pantry and freezer. Rice paper rolls and rice noodle dishes are a major feature, with lots of green leafy vegetables and herbs.

Every recipe is original, created by me as I developed the HUNGER HERO DIET© and lost over 35kg in 35 weeks – without exercise, drugs, or surgery. As I ran the experiment, I painstakingly recorded everything I ate, and photographed every meal. Rest assured that every image in this book is REAL and not photoshopped in any way. What you see is what you get.

The latest scientific evidence was used to select foods that are recognised for their health benefits, but they had to earn their place in the diet by providing the mouth with what it craves – foods with texture and flavour – crunchy, creamy, spicy, savory, salty, and umami.

Foods were included, or omitted, for many reasons, but the end result was a beneficial mix of prebiotics, probiotics, macronutrients (protein, carbs, fats) and micronutrients (vitamins and minerals).

Many foods are repeated over and over, but the reason goes far beyond practicality and monetary economy. If you scroll down the following lists, you will see these foods appearing time and again. They are packed full of vitamins.

Foods containing **water-soluble** vitamins:
- B1 (thiamine): Yeast, pork, cereal grains, sunflower seeds, brown rice, whole-grain rye, asparagus, kale, cauliflower, potatoes, oranges, liver, eggs.
- B2 (riboflavin): Asparagus, bananas, persimmons, okra, silverbeet, cottage cheese, ricotta cheese, milk, yoghurt, steak, eggs, fish, oysters, green beans.
- B3 (niacin): Tuna, beef liver, heart, kidney, chicken, beef, milk, eggs, avocados, dates, tomatoes, leafy greens, broccoli, carrots, sweet potatoes, asparagus, nuts, wholegrains, legumes, mushrooms, yeast.

- B5 (pantothenic acid): Egg yolk, liver, kidney, yeast, meats, wholegrains, broccoli, avocados, royal jelly, roe.
- B6 (pyridoxine): Chickpeas, steak, navy beans, liver, tuna, salmon, chicken breast, bananas, cottage cheese.
- B7 (biotin): Egg yolk, liver, salmon, spinach, broccoli, yoghurt.
- B9 (folic acid): Leafy green vegetables, legumes (beans, lentils), asparagus, spinach, broccoli, avocado, mangoes, lettuce, sweet corn, liver, baker's yeast, sunflower seeds, citrus fruit.
- B12 (cyanocobalamin): Fish, shellfish, meat, poultry, eggs, dairy, and some fortified soy products.
- C (ascorbic acid): Guavas, capsicum, kiwifruit, strawberries, oranges, papayas, broccoli, tomatoes, kale, eggplant, snow peas.

Foods containing **fat-soluble** vitamins:
- A (retinol, carotenoids): Liver, cod liver oil, carrots, broccoli, sweet potato, butter, kale, kiwi fruit, spinach, pumpkin, some cheeses, egg, apricot, cantaloupe melon, and milk. Our bodies convert the beta-carotene into vitamin A.
- D (ergocalciferol): There are traces in salmon, tuna, sardines, oysters, prawns, egg yolks, mushrooms.
- E (tocopherols): Almonds, avocado, eggs, milk, nuts, leafy greens, unheated vegetable oils, wheat germ, wholegrains.
- K (phylloquinone): Leafy greens such as kale, silverbeet, Asian greens, parsley. Vitamin K helps vitamin E with normal blood clotting and wound healing.

How to cook CRISPY SKIN fish

This method for achieving delicious crispy skin and juicy flesh is ideal for cooking any THICK fish fillets WITH THE SKIN ON, especially SALMON, TROUT or BARRAMUNDI.

- Heat pan on high, add drizzle of olive oil, salt, cracked pepper
- If cooking vegetables in the same pan, add them now, and give a little toss.
- Add fish fillet to pan, SKIN SIDE DOWN
- Allow fish to cook until skin becomes crispy. (be patient)
- Drizzle a little oil over the fish, then flip it over
- Using utensils, carefully peel the skin from the fish
- Place the skin in the pan, crispy side up – allowing the fatty side to cook. DO NOT COVER THE PAN
- Season with salt and cracked pepper again
- Leave everything to cook for another minute or so.
- Remove pan from heat and slice cooked fish fillet into goujons (finger-sized strips).

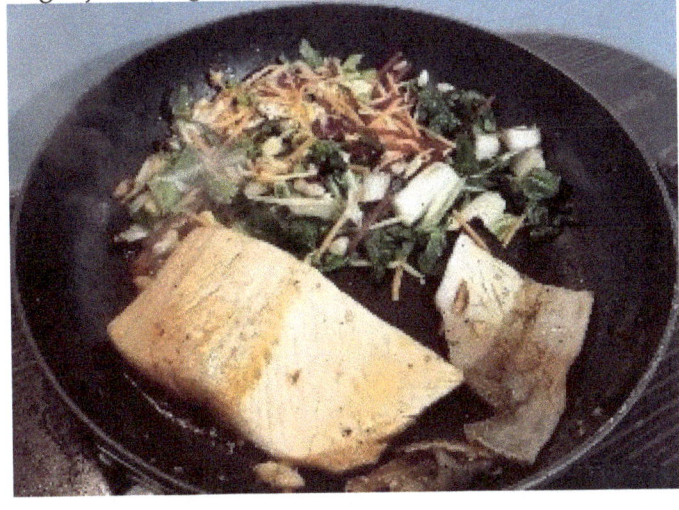

How to PAN-FRY tuna steaks

This method is suitable for firm-fleshed tuna fillets, which can benefit from being cooked as a steak – seared until browned on the outside and medium rare in the middle. Most recipes use individually-wrapped frozen tuna steaks purchased in packs of 10, usually thawed at room temperature before cooking, unless otherwise specified.

- Heat pan on high, add a drizzle of olive oil, salt, cracked pepper, plus a teaspoon of sambal oelek chili paste for extra flavour (if desired)
- If cooking vegetables in the same pan, add them now, and give a little toss.
- Add TUNA STEAK to hot pan
- Cook for a couple of minutes, giving the underside of the tuna a chance to get brown and a little crusty
- Flip the tuna steak (as pictured)
- Leave to cook for another minute or so. You want both sides to be brown and a bit crispy, with a thin line of pink in the middle. If you cook it too long, it becomes dry and tough.
- Remove from pan and slice into finger-sized strips.
- Serve in rice paper rolls, with salad, cooked vegetables, or in a soup broth.

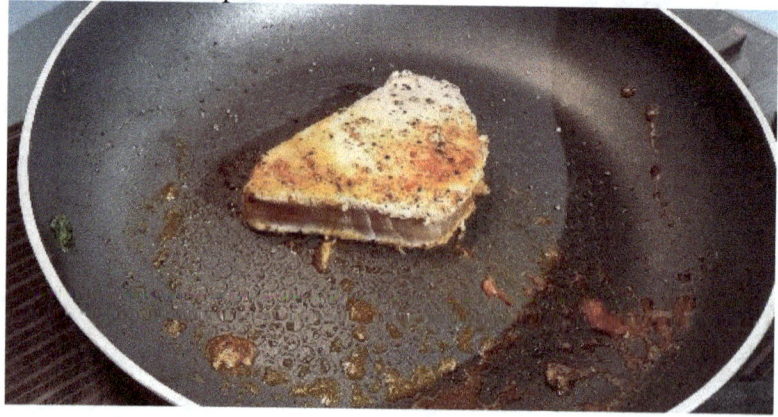

How to PAN-FRY thin fish fillets

This method is suitable for THIN fillets of white fish such as New Zealand HOKI or WHITING, especially when cooked with thin leafy Asian greens, as they have the same cooking time. Most recipes use individually-wrapped frozen fillets, purchased in packs from your supermarket – sometimes thawed in the fridge before cooking, sometimes not, depending on the recipe.

- Heat pan on high, add a drizzle of olive oil, salt, cracked pepper
- If cooking vegetables in the same pan, add them now, and give a little toss.
- Add thawed fish fillet to pan. Cook for a minute or so.
- When the edges of the fish fillet start to turn white, flip the fillet and cook for another minute or so
- Remove pan from heat. Cut into thick strips.

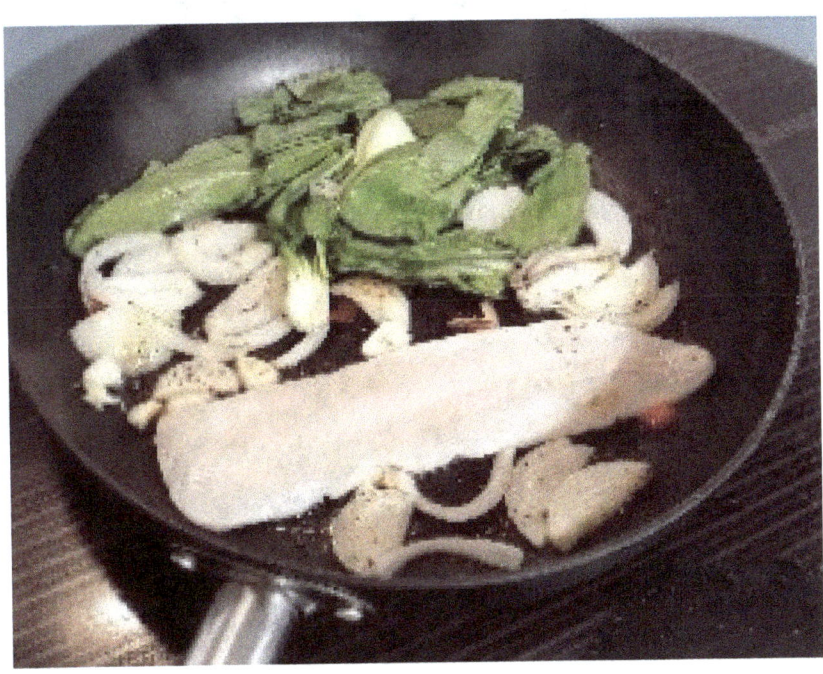

How to STEAM thin fish fillets

This method is suitable for THIN fillets of white fish such as NZ HOKI or WHITING, when cooking with vegetables. Thin fillets can be used fresh, frozen, or thawed.

- Add a drizzle of olive oil to a large pan
- Add a mix of leafy vegetables and give them a stir.
- Place fish fillets on top. Season with salt and pepper
- Cover with a lid. The fish will steam as the veges fry.
- Once the vegetables have softened and the fish has turned opaque white, give everything a gentle toss.
- Remove from heat. Season again.
- Serve with squeeze of lemon, and a dollop of Greek yoghurt.

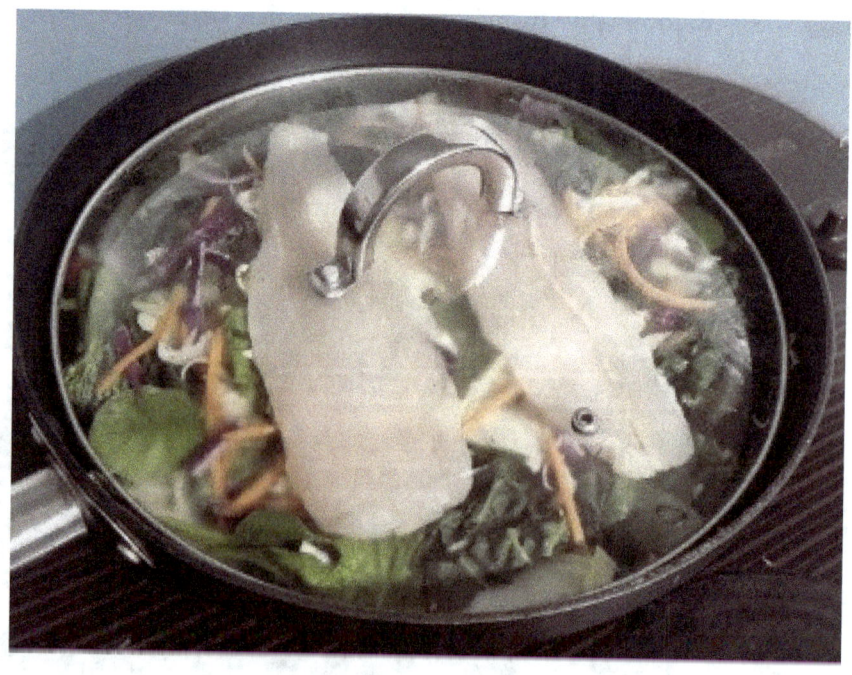

How to BRAISE thick fish fillets

This 2-step method is suitable for any THICK white fish WITHOUT SKIN, such as BARRAMUNDI. If you want to cook it with SKIN ON, follow the recipe for CRISPY SKIN FISH.

- Add a drizzle of olive oil to a large pan
- Add SKINNED side of fish fillet to pan. Season with salt and cracked pepper. A little chopped chili is optional.
- Cook for a couple of minutes
- Flip fish and cook for just a few seconds, then remove partially cooked fish from pan. Set aside on a plate.
- Into the empty pan, add another drizzle of oil
- Add mixed greens, and leave to fry for a minute
- Mix a teaspoon of stock powder into a cup of hot water, pour over vegetables, and give a little stir
- Return the fish to the pan, on top of the vegetables. Cover with lid. Cook for a couple of minutes.
- When vegetables have softened, and fish is opaque (without falling apart), remove from heat. Season again with salt, pepper, and add generous squeeze of lemon. Transfer everything into a serving bowl.

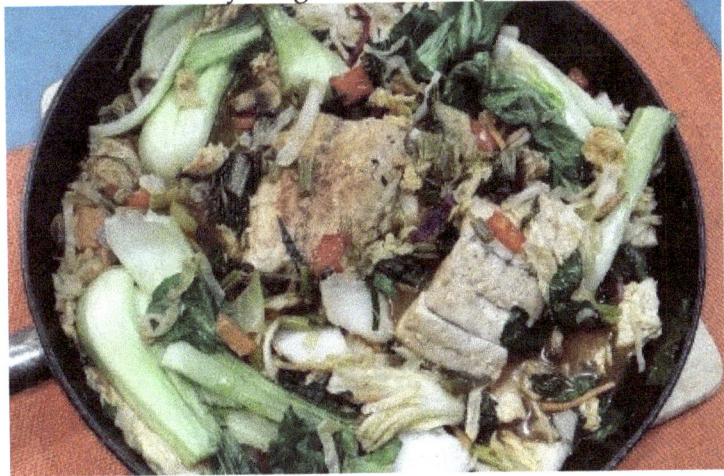

How to make rice paper rolls

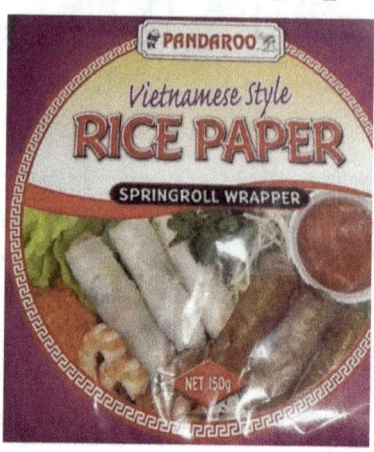

- **Pandaroo Vietnamese Style Rice Paper**, 10 large round sheets per pack

For the weight conscious, these rice paper rounds help maintain correct portion size, and the unique combination of tapioca and rice flours can reduce appetite. When the dry papers are reconstituted in a water bath, the soft pliable wrappers take on a gelatinous feel, and when you eat them, your gut registers a pleasant sense of fullness.

To make our rice paper rolls, you will need a pack of dried rice paper rounds, a serve of protein, creamy Greek yoghurt, sweet and spicy sushi ginger, a touch of chili heat, a cup of mixed coleslaw vegetables (such as cabbage, carrot, celery, onion), a few baby lettuce leaves, some aromatic Asian herbs, and a few slices of avocado when they're in season and not costing a fortune!

These Vietnamese-inspired gluten-free rice paper rolls are a perfect combination of flavours and textures – smooth, chewy, creamy, sour, spicy, crunchy, sweet and aromatic.

They contain all the food groups, with the added benefit of being *prebiotic* (coleslaw) and *probiotic* (natural Greek yoghurt).

METHOD
1. Get organised. Place all ingredients and utensils on a clean kitchen bench. If you can, sit down at the bench too, as this makes it easier to roll the rice papers.
2. Set aside THREE sheets of rice paper (dinner plate size)
3. Place a large flat plate or tray on the bench. Must be large enough to allow for a sheet of rice paper to be submerged in water.
4. Add a little room-temperature tap water to the large plate. (Do not use warm water or the rice paper will soften too quickly.)
5. Submerge one sheet of rice paper in the water. Give it a little poke with your finger to keep it under water for a few seconds. Before it goes limp, lift it out, and lay it flat on a plastic cutting board, or kitchen bench.
6. Quickly build the filling on one side of the wet wrapper, before it becomes too limp to manage. Add wet ingredients first, and finish with dry salad – it acts as a protective cover and makes it less messy to roll up.
7. When you have a little mound of filling neatly arranged on the rice paper, carefully lift the nearest edge and fold over to cover the filling. By starting at the front, you can then fold the sides, and finish by rolling it to the other end. You should have a neat parcel. Repeat.

HINT: Wet rice paper quickly softens to become limp and sticky, so don't be surprised if your first few attempts look untidy. If you make a mess, don't give up; just wrap the whole thing in a large lettuce leaf to hold it together. You will get better with practice, and patience. The trick is to wet one rice paper at a time, get the filling done quickly, and roll it up before the wrapper becomes too soft and sticky.

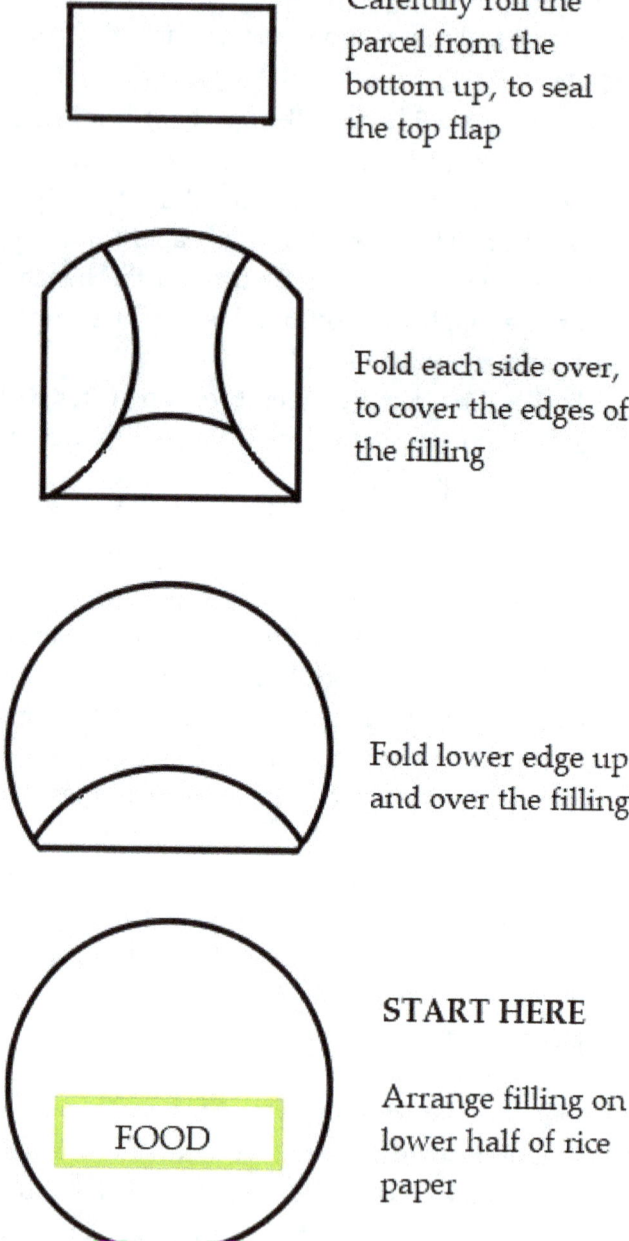

How to prepare rice noodles

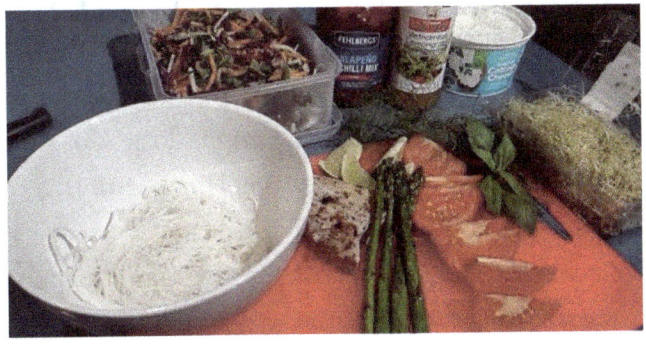

Rice noodles can be a welcome change from rice paper rolls, especially in the winter months when you're wanting a hot plate of food. But don't eat noodles every day if you want to lose weight.

Once you start freewheeling with salads and noodle bowls, you can become heavy handed and extra calories quickly creep into your diet. It is very easy to misjudge quantities, especially noodles, so you need to be very careful if you want to enjoy these delicious variations and continue to lose weight.

Most recipes use reconstituted thin vermicelli rice noodles (hot or cold), while the thicker ribbon noodles are ideal for soups and broths.

Thin vermicelli rice noodles are quick and easy to prepare. Place them in a bowl and cover with boiling water for a few minutes. When soft, drain and put to one side.

When making a noodle soup, you can cheat by dropping the dry vermicelli noodles directly into the hot stock on the stove. This is also the most efficient way to cook thick ribbon noodles. Quick and easy.

So, what does a single serving of noodles look like?

A 500g packet of **Wai Wai Bihoon Rice Vermicelli noodles** contains 10 bundles of dry noodles, each weighing 50g. That's about 180 calories – way too much if you're trying to lose weight or maintain your weight loss. To keep total calories for a meal within appropriate limits, the rice noodle component should not exceed 100 calories.

To achieve this, it's very simple. Take a pair of large kitchen scissors and snip each bundle in half. Store them in a large plastic container. You now have 20 little bundles of noodles, ready to add to your meals.

Flat ribbon noodles are not so quick and easy. But with a little planning, it can be done. Read the label and calculate what a single serve would look like. As with the vermicelli noodles, the packaging on thicker 'rice sticks' or ribbon noodles also recommends 50g as the serving size. But at 180 calories, this is too much. Again, try to limit your serving size to 100 calories.

There are many different brands of thick ribbon rice noodles, but a typical packet weighs 375g, with 8 serves at 50g each. If we reduce serving size to 100 calories, that equates to about 28g per serve, or about 13 serves to a packet of noodles instead of only 8.

There is no way around it. Weigh out 28g of ribbon noodles for an single serve. For efficiency and convenience, I weigh the whole packet into 28g lots, and pop them into resealable sandwich bags. When I'm done, I'll have about 13 little packets, which I then place in a large plastic storage container (with the empty packet, so I know what they are) and store in the pantry until needed. Easy-peasy.

To reconstitute dry thin vermicelli rice noodles

- place a serve of dry vermicelli noodles into a bowl, cover with boiling water, then give a little stir
- Place a lid or plate over the bowl to keep the heat in
- After a few minutes, take a look, and give them a little stir. They should be plump and soft. Drain.
- HINT: If planning to make a soup, don't drain the noodles. Stir in a teaspoon of stock powder (or miso), add some chopped leafy Asian greens, and a few thin slices of a favourite protein. Cover the bowl again for a few minutes to allow the extras to cook, but you can zap in the microwave for a couple of minutes if you want it piping hot. Season to taste.

To reconstitute dry flat ribbon rice noodles

These noodles are thicker than vermicelli, so they need to be cooked in boiling water on the stove for a few minutes.

- Pour a few cups of water into a saucepan, place on the stove, and bring to the boil
- Add a serve of dried flat noodles (make sure there's enough hot water to submerge the noodles). Leave the pan uncovered.
- After a few minutes, take a look, and give a little stir. Remove from stove and drain.
- HINT: If making soup, leave saucepan on stove and don't drain noodles. Stir in a teaspoon of stock powder (or miso), add a handful of chopped leafy greens, and a few thin slices of a favourite protein. Cover and simmer for a couple of minutes. Remove from heat. Pour everything into a soup bowl. Season to taste.

How to add flavour

The recipes in the original HUNGER HERO DIET©, and in this companion series, focus on keeping our mouth happy.

The rough translation for **kuchisabishii** is 'lonely mouth', and this Japanese expression describes why we MINDLESSLY feed our mouths – by smoking, eating, or drinking.

So, to avoid overeating, we need to keep our mouth happy, because a lonely mouth can cause chaos.

It sounds counter-intuitive, but we need to give our mouth what it wants – or at least something that satisfies the specific craving. Those desires might be **textural** (crunchy, crispy, smooth, creamy, liquid, chewy, soft, sticky) or flavourful (sweet, sour, bitter, salty, spicy, savoury/umami).

The major food groups provide most of the textural elements – the seafood proteins, the rice papers rolls and noodles, and the vegetables – and some of the flavours. But most of the flavours will come from things we add, such as cooking sauces and condiments. Here are a few of my favourites, many of which feature in these recipes. You can gain inspiration from what you keep in your fridge door.

Cooking sauces

- Australian or Italian extra virgin olive oil, cold pressed
- **Valcom** Authentic Thai Tom Yum paste (gives a fragrant, spicy chili hit)
- **Valcom** Authentic Thai Pad Thai stir-fry paste (very mild and a little sweet)
- **Jeeny's Oriental Foods** Tamarind Puree, 220g (adds a sour umami-like element to counteract sweetness and adds depth to spicy dishes)

- **Ayam** Vietnamese PHO soup paste
- Malaysian Laksa soup paste
- Tin of **Vegeta** vegetable-flavoured powdered stock
- **Hikari** Japanese Miso Instant Soup with Wakame seaweed, 12 sachets to a pack (a quick way to add depth of flavour to soups)
- Hoisin, Oyster, and Plum sauces
- Passata or pasta sauce
- Light soy sauce and fish sauce can be used to enhance cooking or as a table condiment

Asian condiments

- Iodised salt and freshly-cracked pepper
- A jar of sliced pickled jalapenos
- **Conimex** sambal oelek hot chilli paste
- **Pandaroo** Japanese sweet pickled pink sushi ginger, 200g jar
- **ABC** Kecap Manis sweet soy sauce
- **Chang's** Crispy Noodle Salad Dressing, 280ml (you can taste the hint of sesame oil and soy sauce)
- **Poonsin** Vietnamese dipping sauce for spring rolls, 300ml (goes well with seafood noodle dishes)
- Fresh herbs (Thai basil, Vietnamese mint, dill, fennel)

How to eat the rainbow

The public health message being yelled from rooftops for decades has been, "EAT THE RAINBOW". But most of us either ignore it, or don't fully understand how to do it.

For most of us, vegetables are a chore. We might have a few favourites that we eat regularly, but how many of us eat RED, YELLOW, ORANGE, WHITE, and GREEN on a daily basis? Not many, I'd wager, and not without help.

And if we do think to buy them, they sit in the bottom crisper until they shrivel into nothingness, because we don't know what to do with them, and really couldn't be bothered. Not only is that wasting precious food, but wasting money too.

Then I stumbled across all the pre-cut and pre-packaged SALADS covering numerous shelves in the chilled section of my local supermarket.

Big and small packs of baby salad leaves, some with grated carrot, others with carrot and beetroot. Small packs of finely chopped coleslaw vegetables (cabbage, carrot, celery). And larger packs of coleslaw-type vegetables with varying combinations of popular salad vegetables, with a choice of European or Asian-style dressings.

Once I discovered these, I soon realised how even a subtle change of vegetables or dressings could completely alter the flavour profile of a salad. Most contained some type of shredded cabbage (European green, red, or Asian wombok), with shredded carrot, sliced onion, chopped shallots, and celery. Others had variations like grated raw beetroot, corn kernels, or Mizuna lettuce. Without realising it, I was EATING THE RAINBOW, and loving it.

I had thought these packs were an expensive indulgence, but then I realised how far one pack could stretch. After a few days of adding fresh salad vegetables to meals, I added the remaining bits to whatever I was cooking, even the salad greens! Now I do this all the time, and good food was never so easy.

These salad packs feature as a core element in recipes in this book, and in THE HUNGER HERO DIET©.

They add textural crunch to our meals, help us to get the nutrition we need by EATING THE RAINBOW, and we stop wasting food and money buying vegetables we forget to eat.

These are some of the amazing salad packs I've enjoyed at different times throughout the year. I suggest starting with a basic coleslaw mix, such as the Crunchy Noodle Coleslaw kit, then experiment by mixing them around. Every major supermarket has a selection, but these are from my local:

- Woolworth's Crunchy Noodle Coleslaw Kit
- Woolworth's Slaw Kits, Creamy Classic Coleslaw Kit,
- Woolworth's Classic Coleslaw
- Woolworth's Fine Cut Coleslaw
- Woolworth's Four Seasons Coleslaw
- Woolworth's Slaw Kits Kaleslaw
- Woolworth's Asian Style Salad Kit
- Woolworth's Thai Salad Kit.

By the way, most salad packs contain extra sachets of creamy salad dressings and other bits. These are extra calories you don't need. Only keep a couple in the kitchen door for occasional use, or when a recipe suggests you use them. Bin the rest.

TUNA STEAKS

Tuna is an excellent source of protein, omega-3s, phosphorous, and vitamins B3, B12 and D. Yellowfin tuna is a rich source of selenium – which helps reduce inflammation and oxidative stress (free radicals).

- **Ocean Chef** Yellowfin Tuna Steaks (10 wrapped frozen portions per 1kg pack) from Woolworths supermarkets

Take a single portion out of the freezer and leave in the fridge to thaw during the day, or just leave it out on the kitchen sink for an hour before you need it.

When thawed, pan fry for a couple of minutes either side in a non-stick pan with some chopped up veg and you're done. A little cracked pepper, drizzle of olive oil, and there's dinner. Too easy! You don't have to be a good cook to eat well. Cook it to medium-rare or medium, even well-done if you must; it's very forgiving.

But never overcook fresh tuna. If lucky enough to find fresh tuna steaks, use the absolute minimum cooking time. Make the most of its silky texture and delicate flavour. Rare to medium-rare is ideal.

Frozen tuna is much more robust, and the packs in the supermarket make it very affordable.

1. Tuna rolls, fennel, jalapenos

- Pan-fried tuna steak, sliced
- 3 rice paper rounds
- Pickled pink sushi ginger, jalapenos
- Southern-style coleslaw kit with spicy dressing
- Grated fennel bulb
- Vietnamese mint, coriander
- Dried onion flakes sprinkled across the top

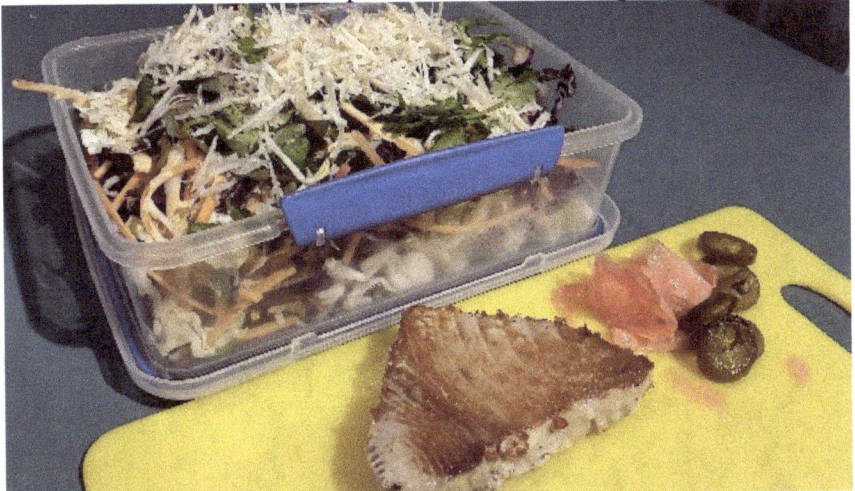

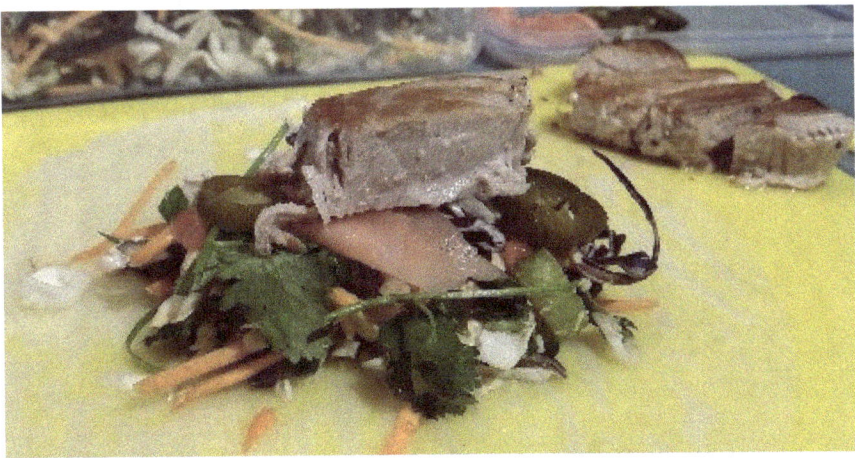

2. Tuna rolls, chili, cranberry sauce

- Pan-fried tuna steak, sliced
- 3 rice paper rounds
- Fresh chili, chopped
- Dollop of Greek yoghurt in each roll
- Cup of Crunchy Coleslaw salad kit (dry)
- Cranberry sauce

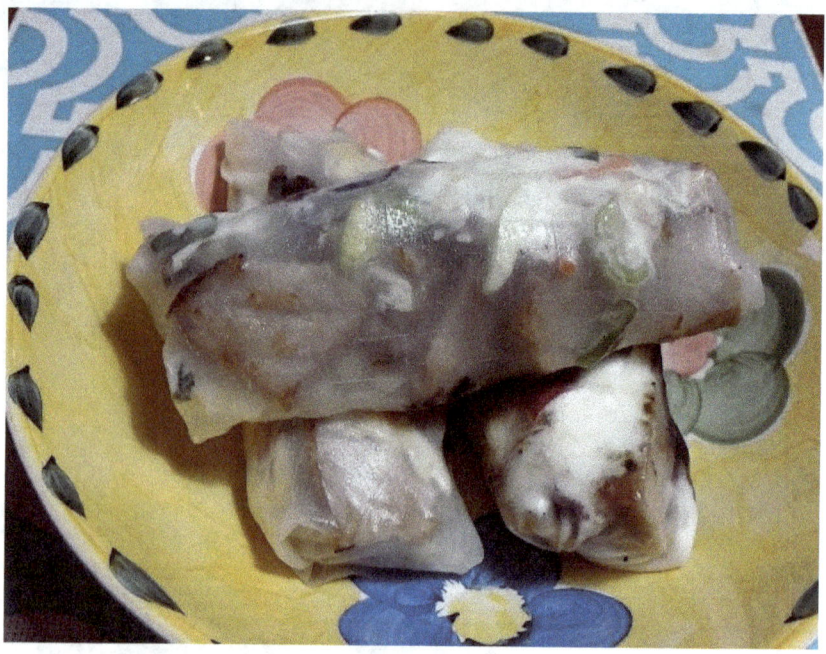

3. Tuna rolls, fresh ginger, basil

- Pan-fried tuna steak, sliced
- 3 rice paper rounds
- Teaspoon grated fresh ginger
- Dollop of Greek yoghurt in each roll
- Cup of mixed coleslaw/kaleslaw salad kit
- Thai basil

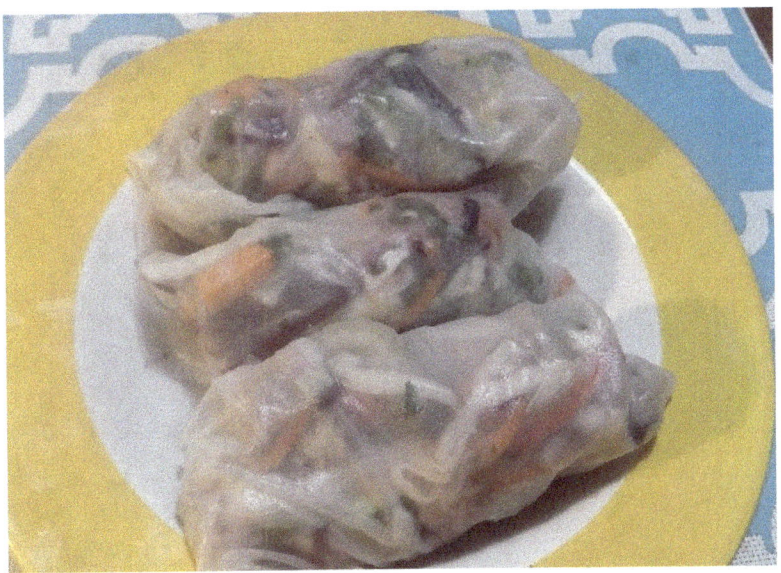

4. Tuna rolls, avo, sambal oelek

- Pan-fried tuna steak, sliced
- 3 rice paper rounds
- Pickled pink sushi ginger
- Greek yoghurt
- ¼ avocado
- Teaspoon sambal oelek chili paste
- Cup of Southern Coleslaw salad (dry)

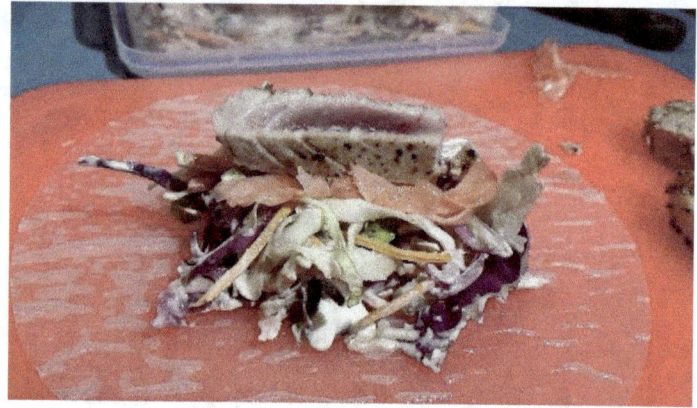

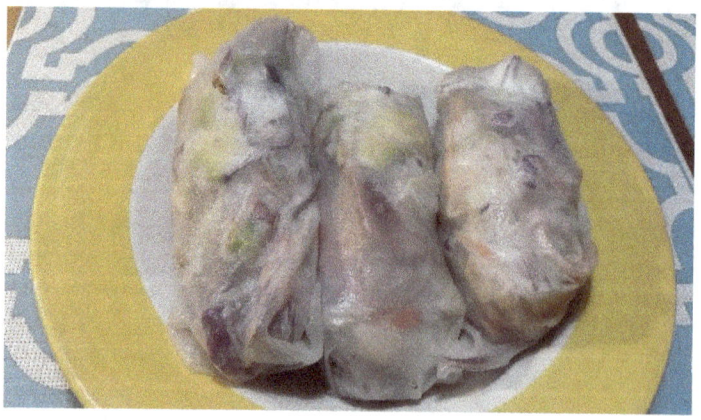

5. Tuna rolls, avo, lemon juice

- Pan-fry thawed tuna steak in olive oil, cracked pepper
- 3 rice paper rounds
- Greek yoghurt
- ¼ avocado
- Cup of coleslaw with dressing
- Lemon juice

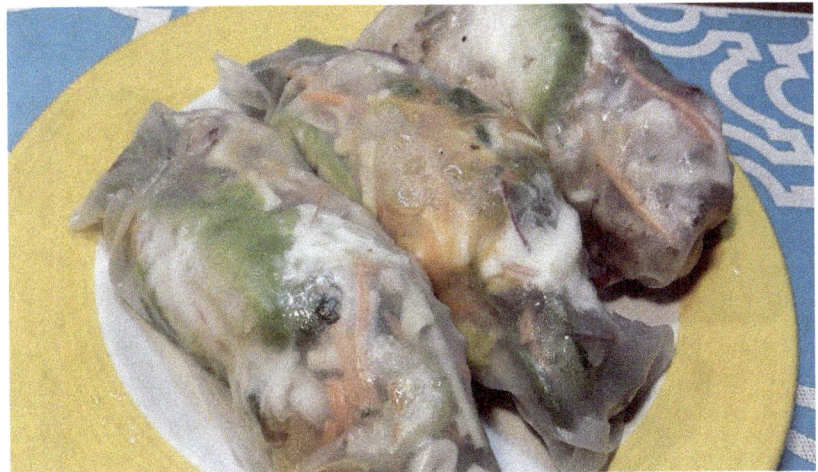

6. Tuna rolls, tahini, black olives

- Heat pan on high, add drizzle of olive and sesame oils, teaspoon sambal oelek, salt, cracked pepper
- Add thawed tuna steak to hot pan
- Cook on one side for a couple of minutes
- Flip and cook on other side.
- Remove from pan, slice, allow to cool a little.

Make rice paper rolls with sliced tuna:
- Cup of mixed coleslaw
- Cup of baby leaf salad
- Greek yoghurt, tahini, black olives.

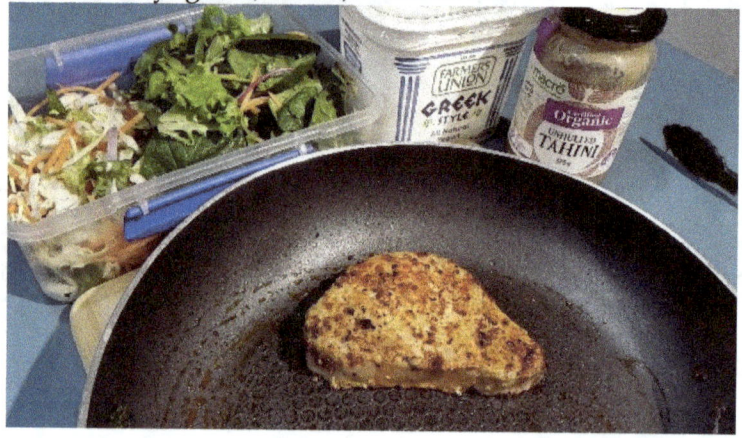

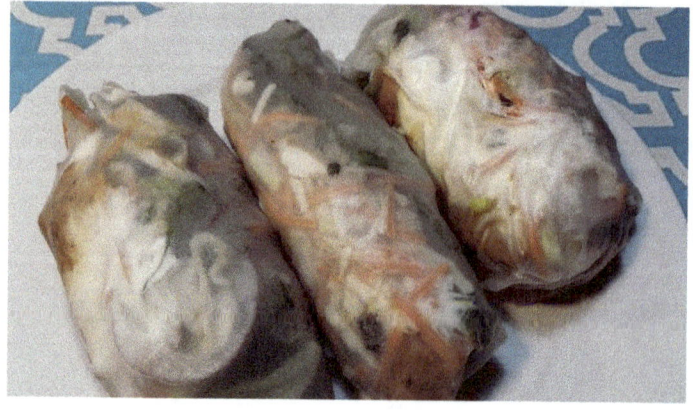

7. Tuna rolls, avo, jalapenos

- Pan-fried tuna steak, sliced
- 3 rice paper rounds
- Pickled pink sushi ginger
- ½ avocado
- Cup of mixed coleslaw/kaleslaw (dry)

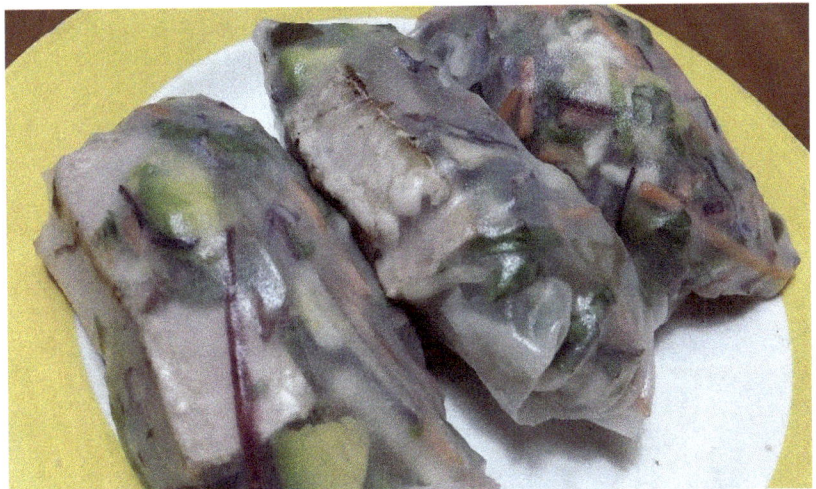

8. Tuna rolls, medium rare, pineapple

- Pan-fry FRESH tuna steak in olive with broccolini
- Season and cook until tuna MEDIUM RARE, then slice.

Make rolls
- 3 rice paper rounds
- Pickled pink sushi ginger, jalapenos
- Greek yoghurt, ¼ avocado
- Sliced fresh pineapple
- Cup of mixed kaleslaw salad (dry) with sliced red onion
- Alfalfa sprouts, dill
- Serve tuna rolls with broccolini on the side

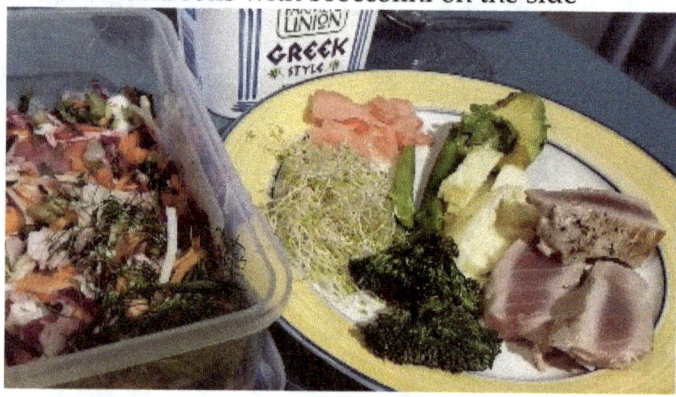

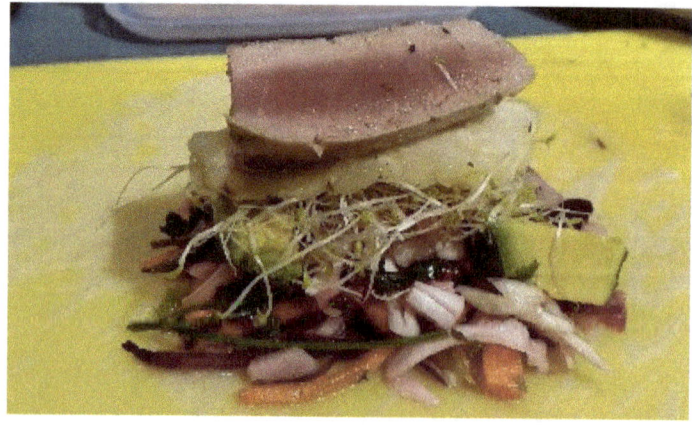

9. Tuna rolls, nori, Asian salad

- 3 rice paper rounds
- Pan-fried tuna steak, sliced
- Pickled sushi ginger
- Dollop of Greek yoghurt in each roll
- Asian salad kit, with dressing
- ½ sheet nori seaweed, snipped into small pieces
- Vietnamese mint, coriander

Make with half the tuna inside the rolls, and the rest served on top.

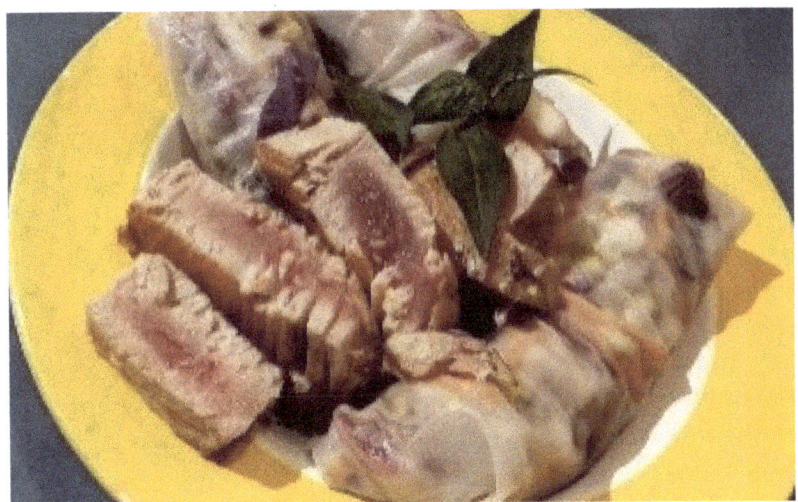

10. Tuna rolls, jalapenos, coleslaw

- Pan-fried tuna steak, sliced
- 3 rice paper rounds
- Greek yoghurt
- Jalapenos
- Cup of Crunchy Coleslaw salad (dry)
- Lettuce leaves

Make with half the tuna inside the rolls, and the rest served on top.

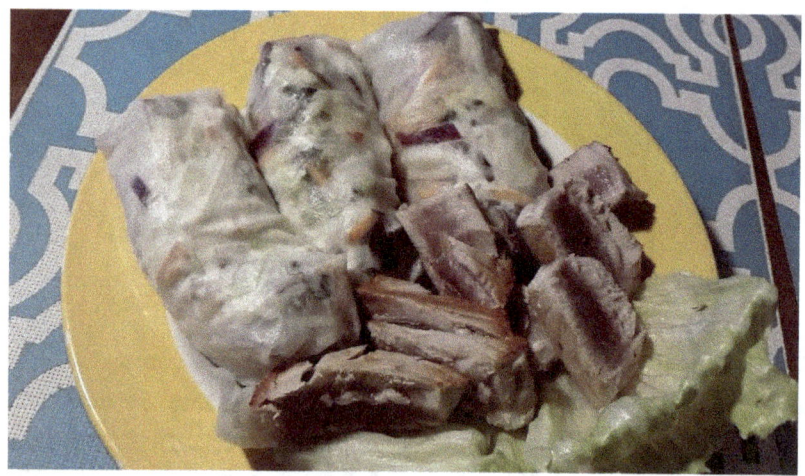

11. Rare tuna rolls, coleslaw, ginger

- Sear both sides of a tuna steak in a hot pan with olive oil, thinly slice

   Make rolls
- 3 rice paper rounds
- Pickled pink sushi ginger
- Greek yoghurt
- Cup of mixed coleslaw/kaleslaw (dry)

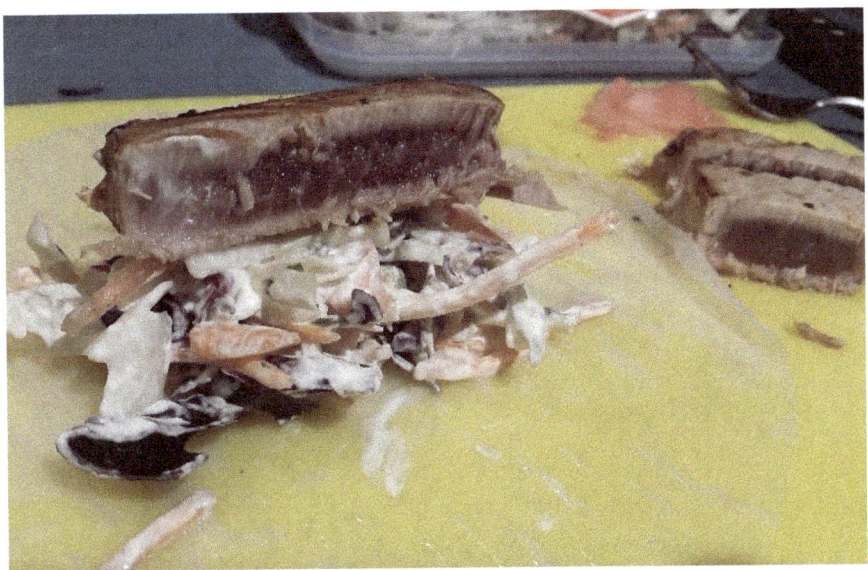

12. Rare tuna rolls, sesame, balsamic

- Quickly sear tuna steak in very hot pan, with olive oil, sesame oil, balsamic vinegar
- 3 rice paper rounds
- Greek yoghurt
- Cup of mixed coleslaw (dry)
- drizzle of Vietnamese Dipping Sauce for Spring Rolls

Make with half the tuna inside the rolls, and the rest served on top.

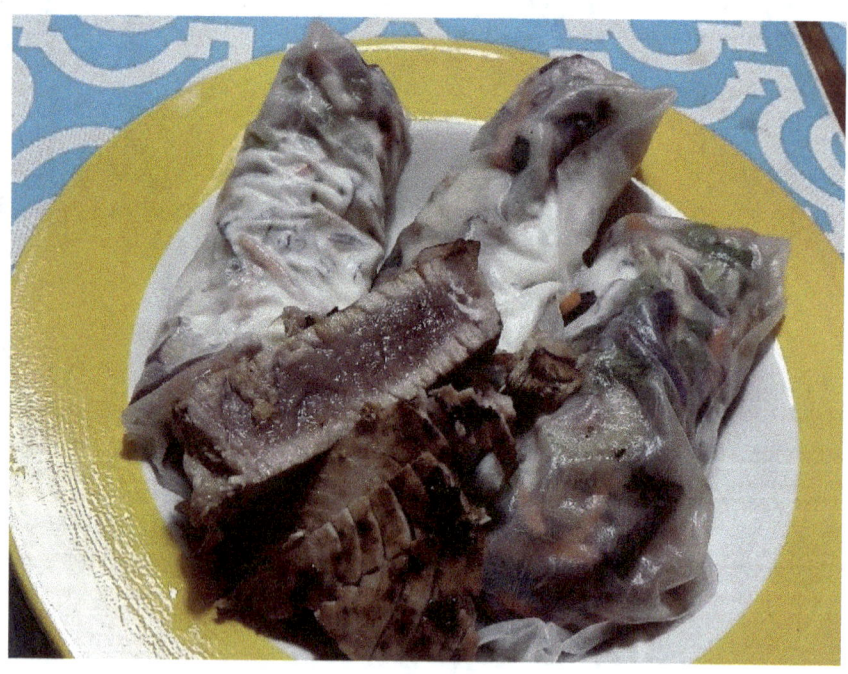

13. Balsamic salad rolls, with tuna

- Pan-fry thawed tuna steak in olive oil, salt, cracked pepper
- 3 rice paper rounds
- Jalapenos
- Greek yoghurt
- Cup of mixed coleslaw (dry)

Make vegetable rolls, top with sliced tuna steak, then drizzle with balsamic vinegar.

Messy and unconventional, but delicious.

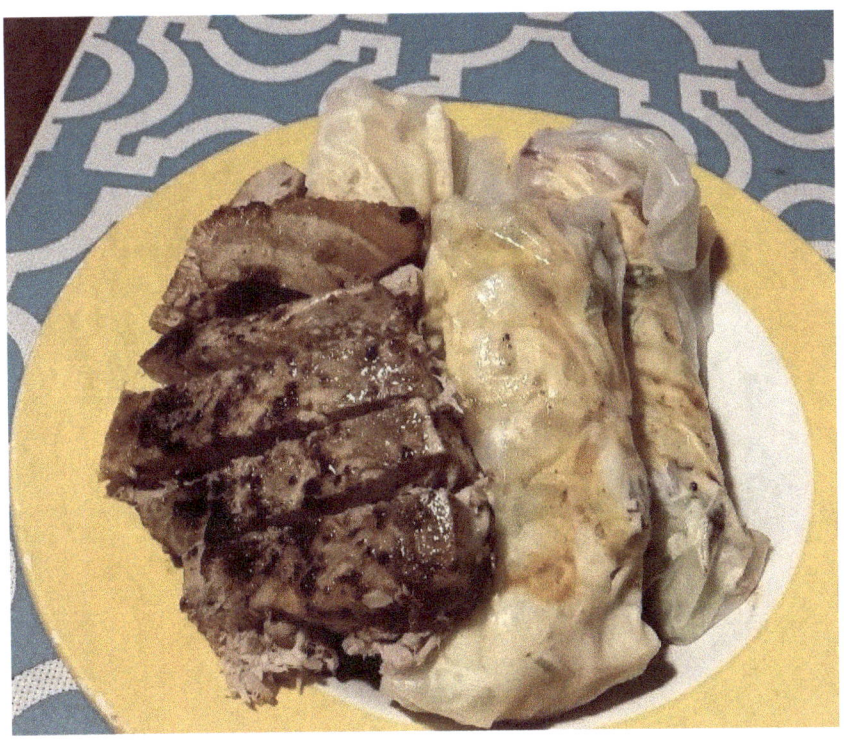

14. Coleslaw rolls, spicy tuna

- Pan-fry thawed tuna steak in olive oil, cracked pepper, sambal oelek
- 3 rice paper rounds
- Pickled sushi ginger
- Jalapenos
- Dollop of Greek yoghurt in each roll
- Cup of crunchy coleslaw with dressing
- Shredded iceberg lettuce

Make vegetable rolls, then serve sliced tuna on top. Season with salt.

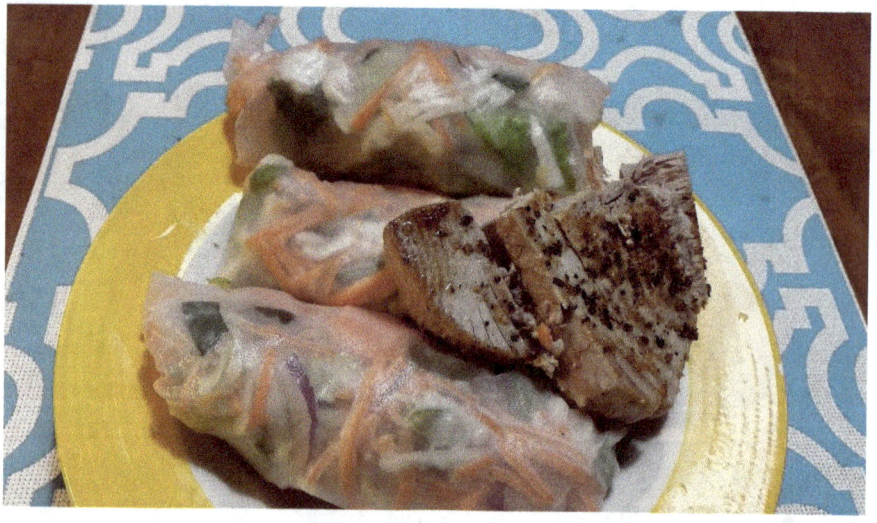

15. Coleslaw rolls, cranberry, tuna

- Pan-fried tuna steak, sliced
- 3 rice paper rounds
- Pickled pink sushi ginger
- Jalapenos
- Greek yoghurt
- Cranberry sauce
- Cup of mixed coleslaw (dry)
- Shredded iceberg lettuce
- Vietnamese Dipping Sauce

Make vegetable rolls, top with sliced tuna steak, then drizzle with Vietnamese Dipping Sauce.

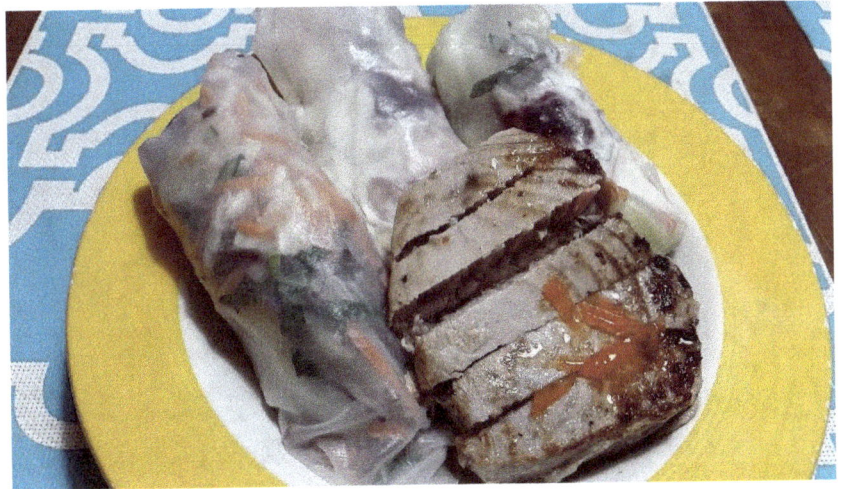

16. Asian salad rolls, crispy tuna

- Pan-fried tuna steak until crispy, then sliced
- 3 rice paper rounds
- Pickled pink sushi ginger
- Jalapenos
- Greek yoghurt
- ¼ avocado
- Cup of Asian coleslaw mix (dry)

Make vegetable rolls, top with sliced tuna steak, then drizzle with Vietnamese Dipping Sauce.

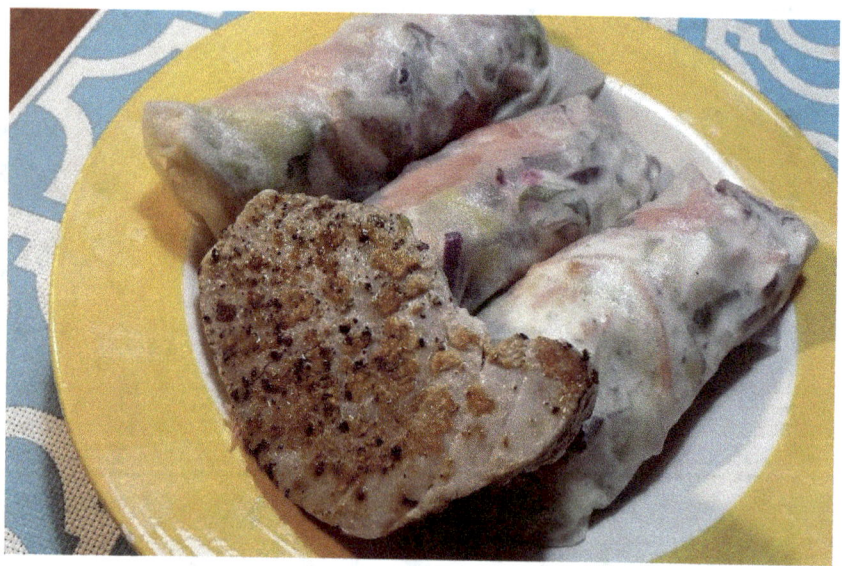

17. Coleslaw rolls, avo, chili tuna

- Pan-fried tuna steak in olive oil, chili, salt, cracked pepper, then sliced
- 3 rice paper rounds
- ½ avocado
- Cup of coleslaw/kaleslaw mix (dry)
- Drizzle of green Asian Seafood sauce and Vietnamese Dipping sauce

Make vegetable rolls, top with sliced tuna steak, then drizzle with the Asian sauces.

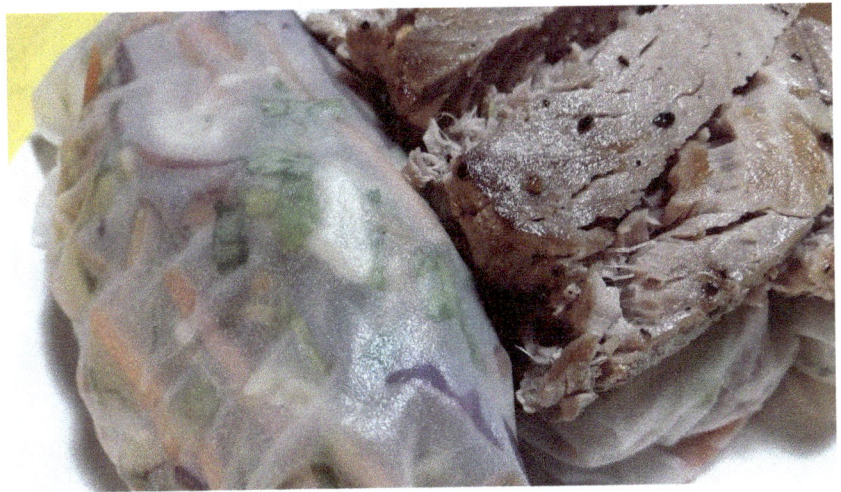

18. Coleslaw rolls, avo, crispy tuna

- Pan-fried crispy tuna steak, cracked pepper, then sliced
- 3 rice paper rounds
- Pickled pink sushi ginger
- ½ avocado
- Cup of coleslaw/kaleslaw mix (dry)
- Cup of mixed baby leaves

Make vegetable rolls, top with sliced tuna steak, then drizzle with the Asian sauces.

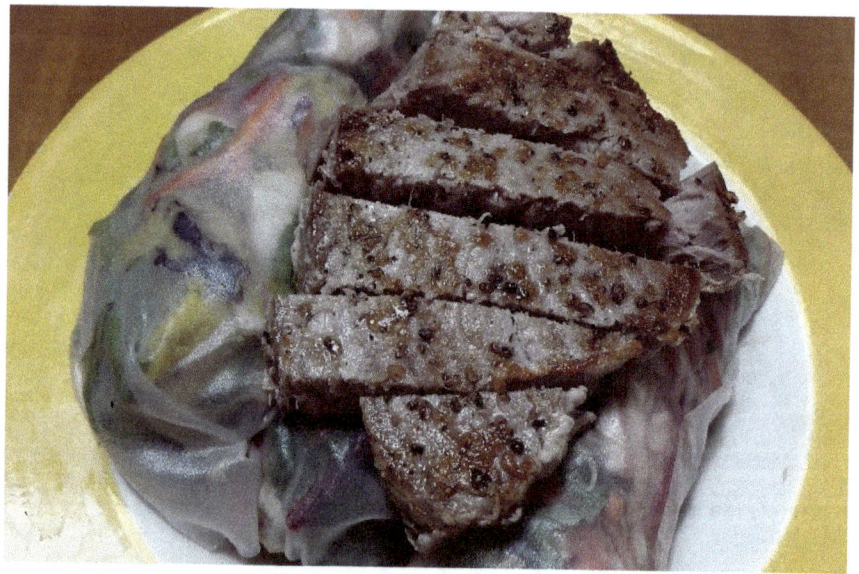

19. Coleslaw rolls, tuna, asparagus

- Pan-fry tuna steak in olive oil with asparagus. Season.
- Cook until tuna is MEDIUM, slice.

Make rolls
- 3 rice paper rounds
- Pickled pink sushi ginger, jalapenos
- Greek yoghurt
- Cup of mixed coleslaw salad (dry) with sliced red onion
- Shredded iceberg lettuce
- Lemon juice

Make vegetable rolls, top with sliced tuna steak and asparagus. Squeeze of lemon juice.

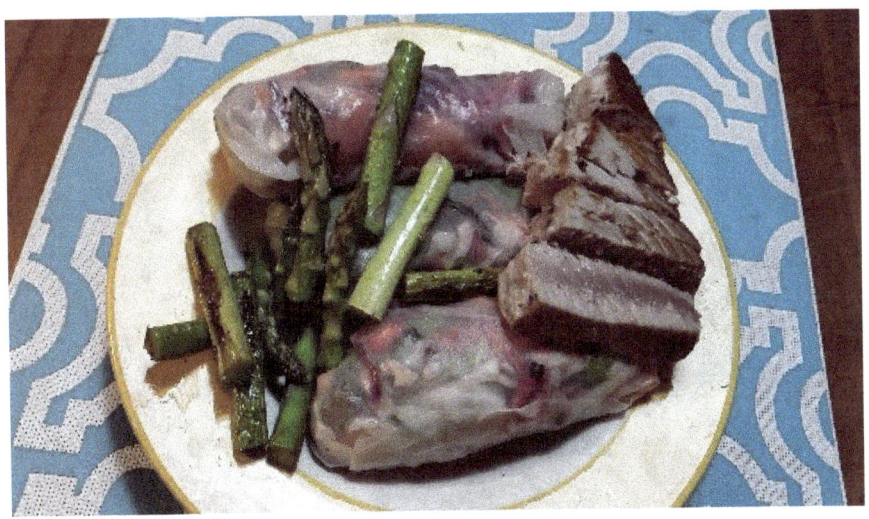

20. Tuna rolls, Asian greens, herbs

- Pan-fry tuna in olive oil, with Asian greens
- Season with salt and cracked pepper

Make rolls
- 3 rice paper rounds
- Pickled pink sushi ginger
- ¼ avocado
- Greek yoghurt
- Cup of mixed coleslaw (dry)
- Chili, Viet mint, coriander, fennel herb

Make with half the tuna inside the rolls, and the rest served on side with Asian greens.

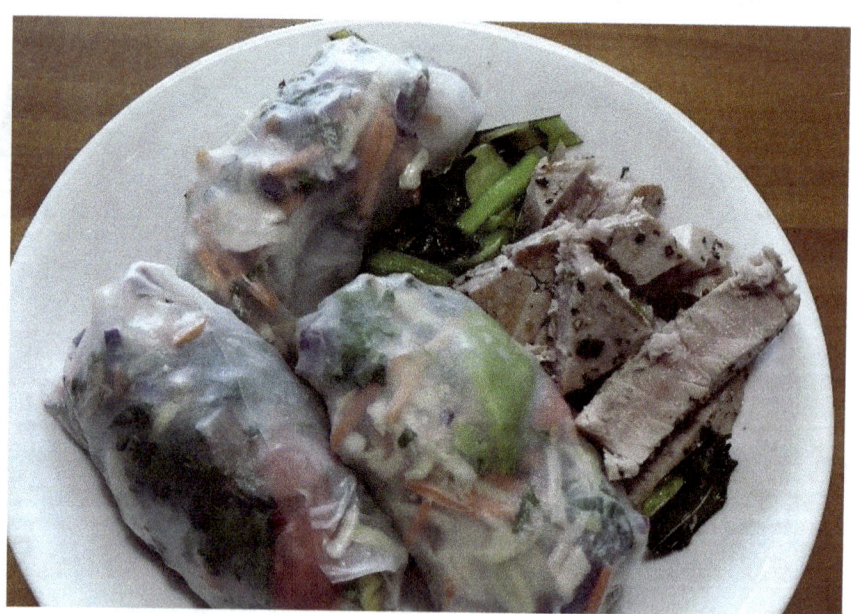

21. Tuna rolls, cottage cheese, silverbeet

- Pan-fry tuna in olive oil, with chopped silverbeet
- Season with salt, cracked pepper, lemon juice
  Make rolls
- 3 rice paper rounds
- Pickled pink sushi ginger
- Jalapenos
- 2 tablespoons of Creamed cottage cheese
- Cup of coleslaw (dry)

Make with half the tuna inside the rolls, and the rest served on side with greens.

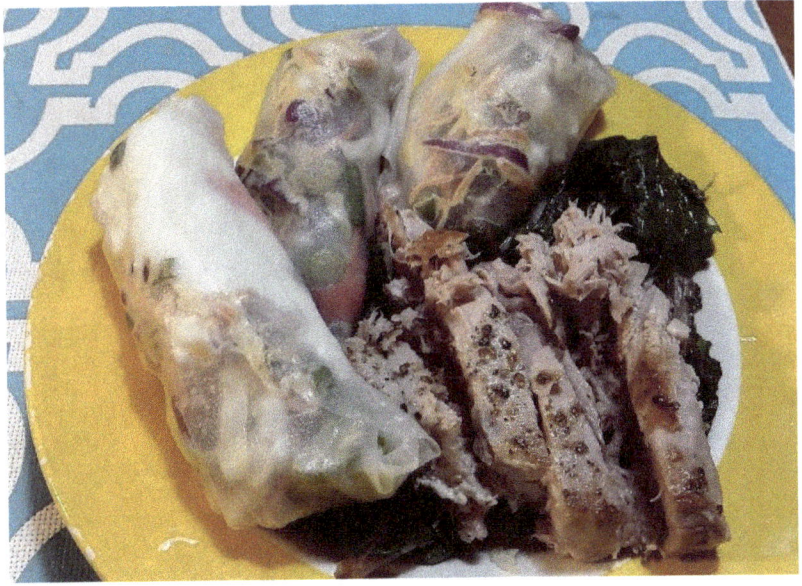

22. Sesame tuna rolls, asparagus, bok choy

- Pan-fry tuna in olive and sesame oils
- Add bok choy and asparagus
- Season with salt and cracked pepper.

Make rolls
- 3 rice paper rounds
- Pickled pink sushi ginger, sambal oelek chili paste
- Greek yoghurt, ¼ avocado
- Cup of mixed kaleslaw salad kit (dry)
- Thai basil, Viet mint, parsley, fennel, lime juice

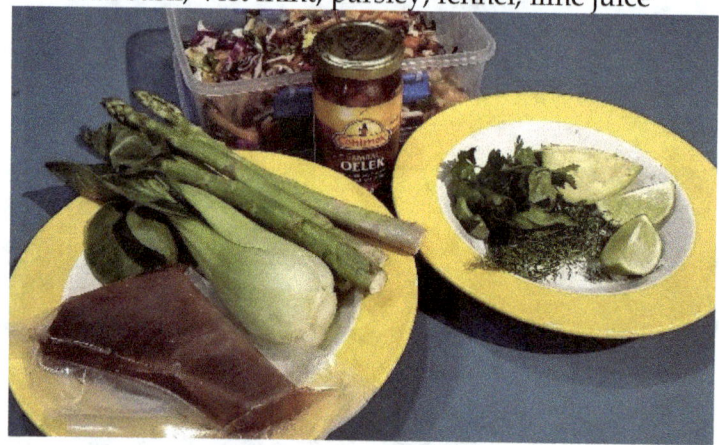

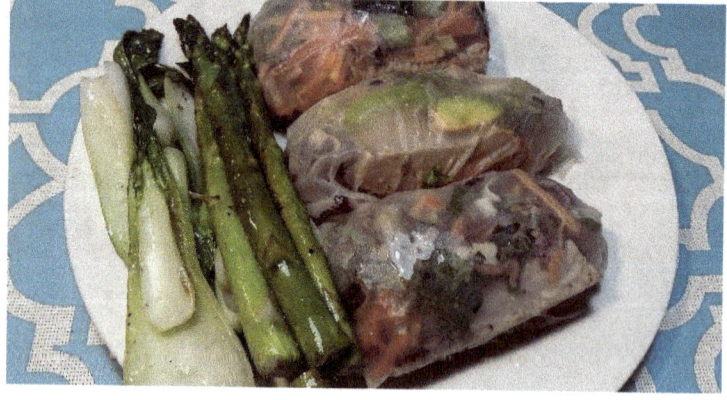

23. Tuna rolls, broccolini, fennel

- Pan-fry tuna steak in oil with broccolini
- 3 rice paper rounds
- Pickled pink sushi ginger, jalapenos
- Sambal oelek, lime juice
- Southern-style coleslaw kit with spicy dressing
- Grated fennel bulb
- Vietnamese mint, coriander

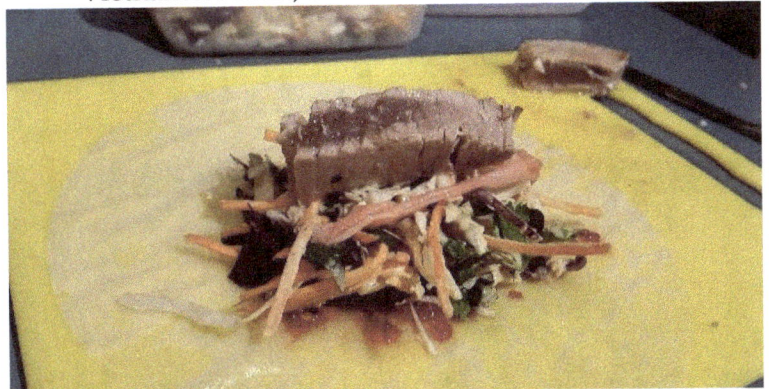

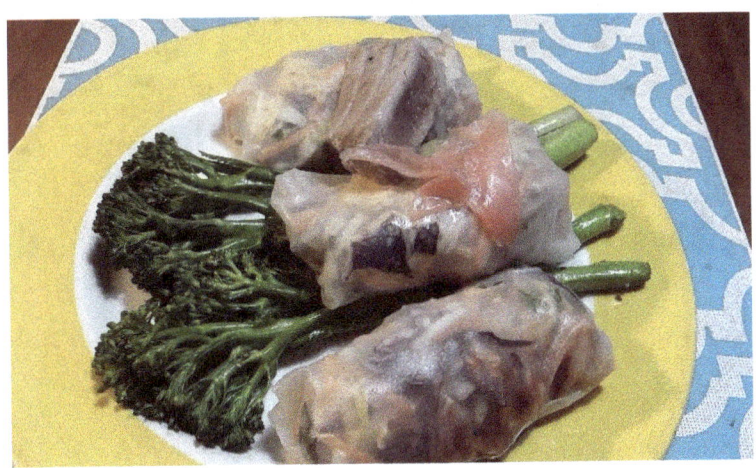

24. Green chili tuna rolls, nori, broccolini

- Pan-fry tuna in olive oil, with salt, cracked pepper
- Add chopped green chili, broccolini
- When cooked, take off the heat and slice tuna

Make rolls
- 3 rice paper rounds
- Greek yoghurt
- ½ sheet nori seaweed
- Cup of mixed coleslaw/kaleslaw salad kit (dry)
- Vietnamese Lemongrass Dressing

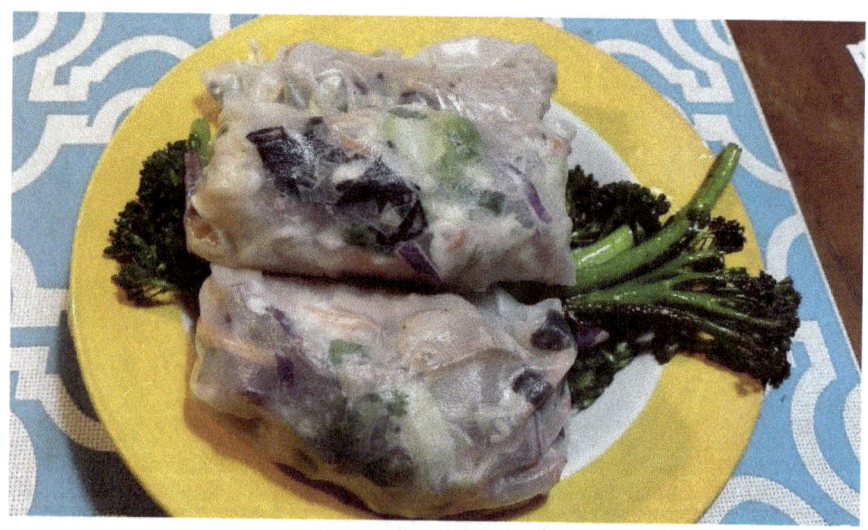

25. Chili tuna rolls, Caesar dressing

- Pan-fry tuna in olive oil, with salt, cracked pepper
- Add chopped chili, asparagus spears
- When cooked, take off the heat and slice tuna

Make rolls
- 3 rice paper rounds
- Caesar Salad Dressing
- Cup of mixed coleslaw/kaleslaw salad kit (dry)

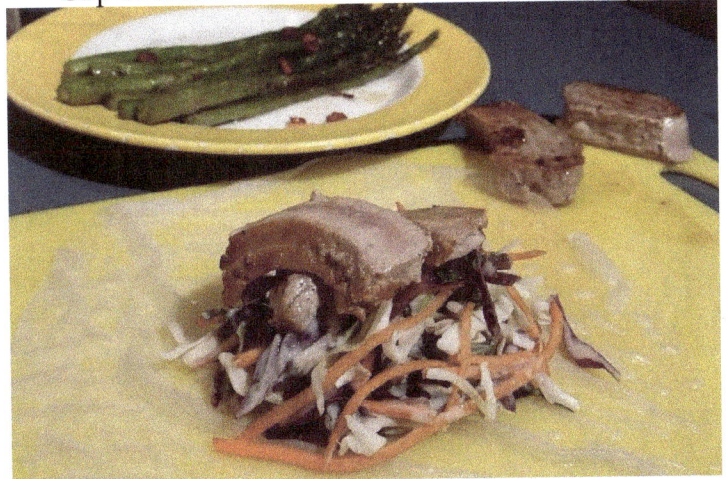

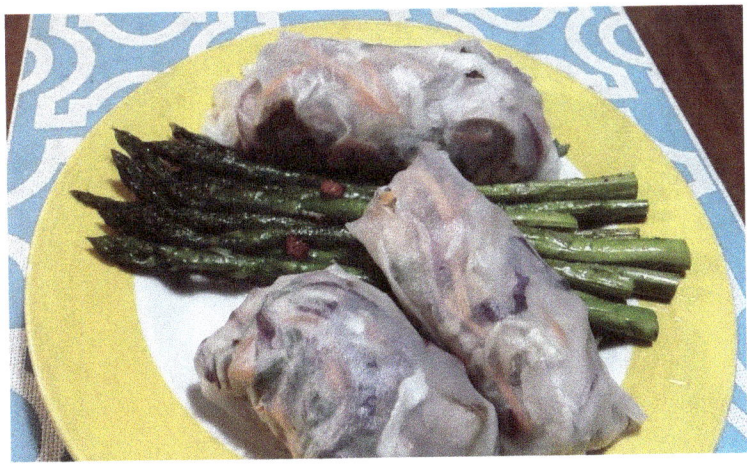

26. Chili tuna rolls, asparagus, spicy dressing

- Pan-fry tuna in olive oil, with salt, cracked pepper
- Add chopped chili, asparagus spears
- When cooked, take off the heat and slice tuna

Make rolls
- 3 rice paper rounds
- Pickled pink sushi ginger
- Cup of Southern Coleslaw salad kit, with spicy dressing

Serve with asparagus on the side.

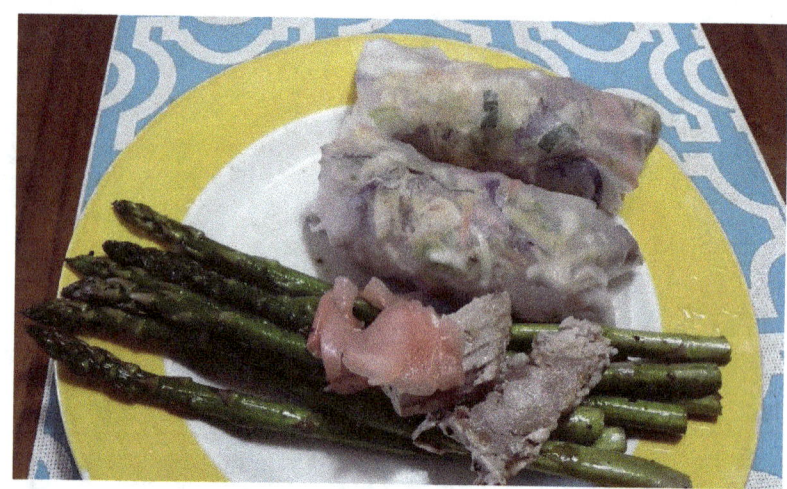

27. Green chili tuna rolls, pineapple

- Pan-fry tuna in olive oil, salt, cracked pepper
- Add chopped green chili, pineapple, broccolini
- When cooked, take off the heat and slice tuna

Make rolls
- 3 rice paper rounds
- Pickled pink sushi ginger
- Pickled red onion
- Greek yoghurt
- Cup of mixed coleslaw/kaleslaw salad kit (dry)
- Serve with fresh lemon wedges

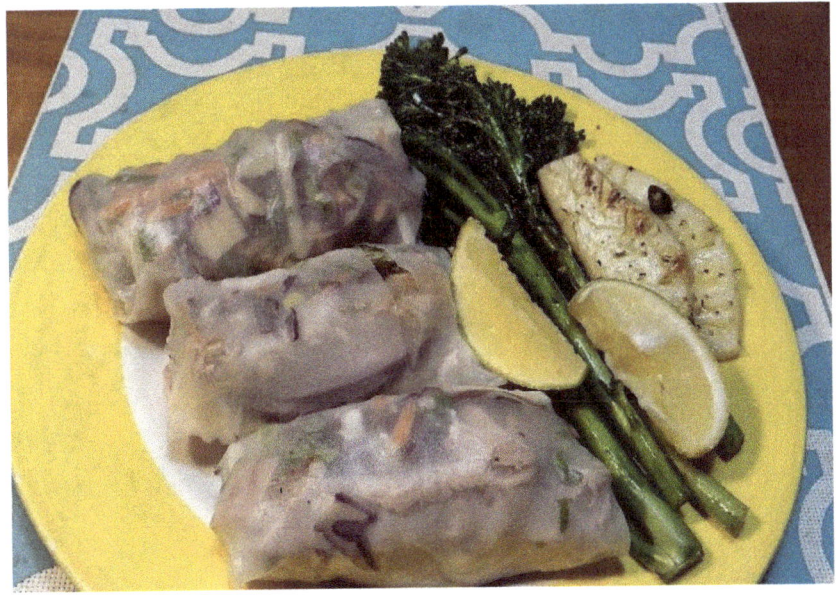

28. Chili tuna rolls, fried greens

- Pan-fry tuna in olive oil, chili, salt, cracked pepper
- Add chopped silverbeet, broccolini
- When cooked, take off the heat and slice tuna

Make rolls
- 3 rice paper rounds
- Pickled pink sushi ginger
- ¼ avocado
- Greek yoghurt
- Cup of mixed coleslaw salad kit (dry)
- Serve with fresh lemon wedges

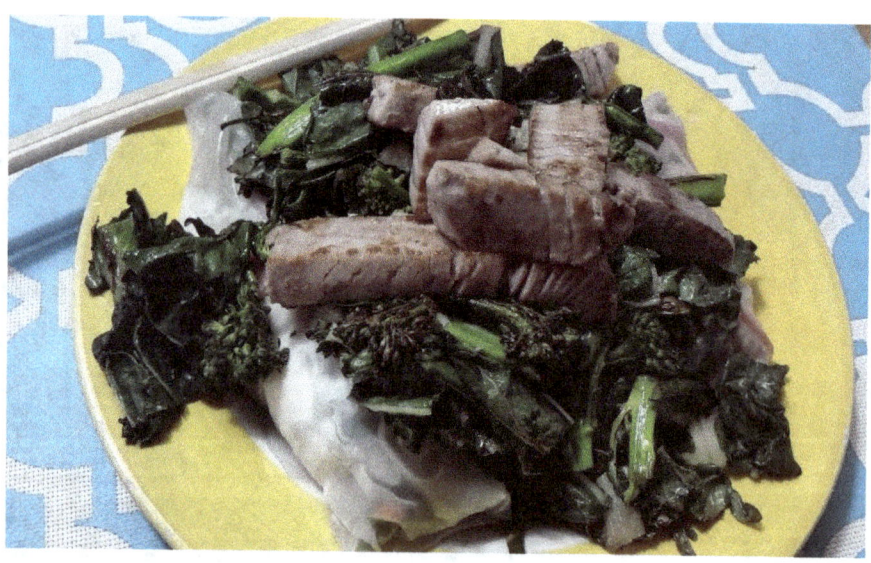

29. Guacamole salad rolls, chili tuna

- Pan-fry tuna in olive oil, salt, cracked pepper
- Add chopped red chili, broccolini
- When cooked, take off the heat and slice tuna

For guacamole dip, mix together

- ¼ avocado
- ½ cup Greek yoghurt
- Teaspoon sambal oelek chili paste
- Season with salt, pepper

Make salad rolls

- 3 rice paper rounds
- Pickled pink sushi ginger
- Guacamole dip
- Cup of mixed coleslaw/kaleslaw salad kit (dry)
- Vietnamese mint
- Serve sliced tuna and fried broccolini on the side.

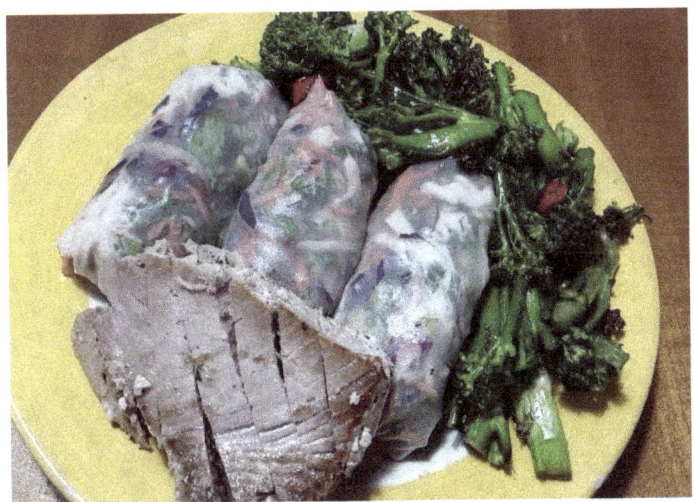

30. Pan-fried tuna, tomato, pepita, salad

- Dry pan-fry tuna steak in hot pan (without oil)
- Season with salt, pepper
- Add a tablespoon of pepitas and sesame seeds, and gently stir across the heated pan. (A little pack of seeds comes in one of the coleslaw salad kits.)

Salad bowl
- Baby salad leaves
- Mixed coleslaw/kaleslaw, with coleslaw dressing
- Fresh tomato wedges
- Add sliced tuna and roasted seeds
- Top with chopped herbs (fennel, Vietnamese mint)
- Drizzle balsamic or apple cider vinegar on tomatoes.

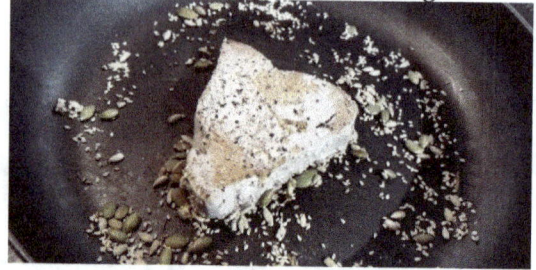

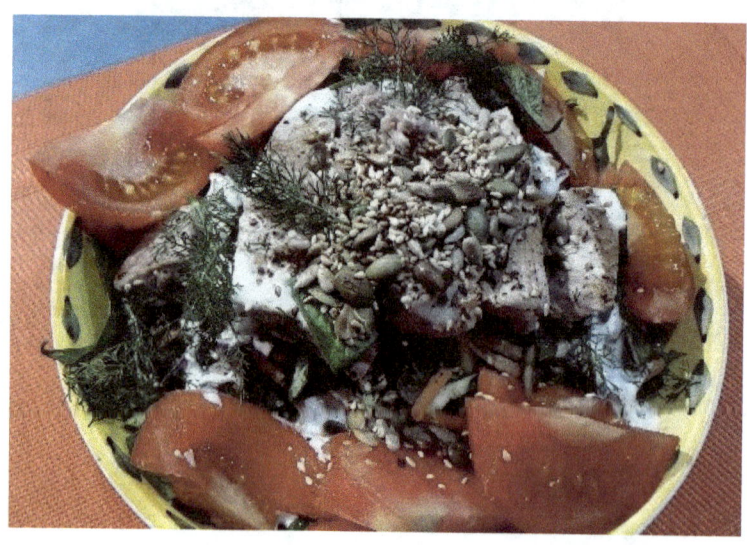

31. Pan-fried tuna, asparagus, salad bowl

- Pan-fry tuna steak in olive oil, sambal oelek
- Add chopped asparagus, salt, pepper
  In serving bowl
- Add cup of crunchy coleslaw, with spicy dressing
- ¼ avocado
- Top with sliced tuna, asparagus, squeeze of lemon

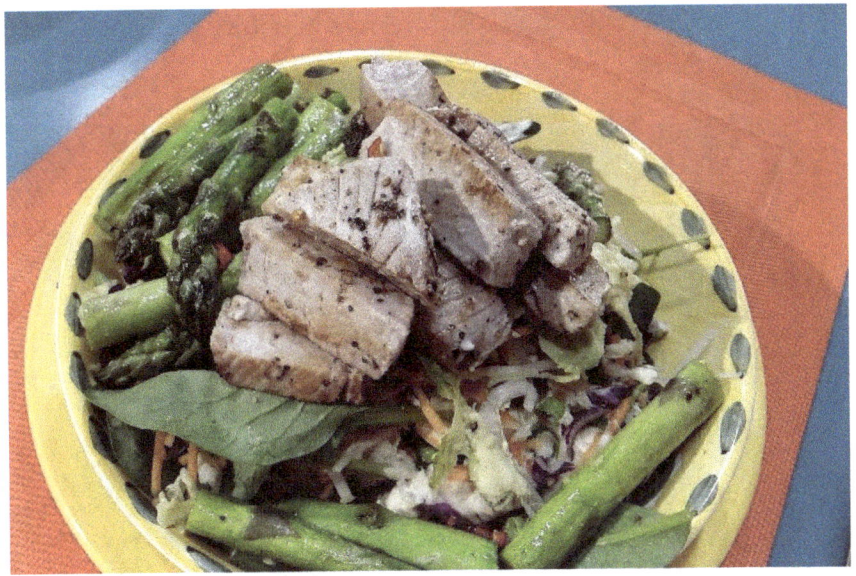

32. Pan-fried tuna, silverbeet, asparagus

Simple but delicious.

- Pan-fry thawed tuna in hot pan with olive oil
- Season with salt, cracked pepper
- Add chopped silverbeet
- Add chopped asparagus
- Transfer vegetables to a dinner plate
- Place tuna on top
- Serve with squeeze of fresh lemon juice
- Season to taste.

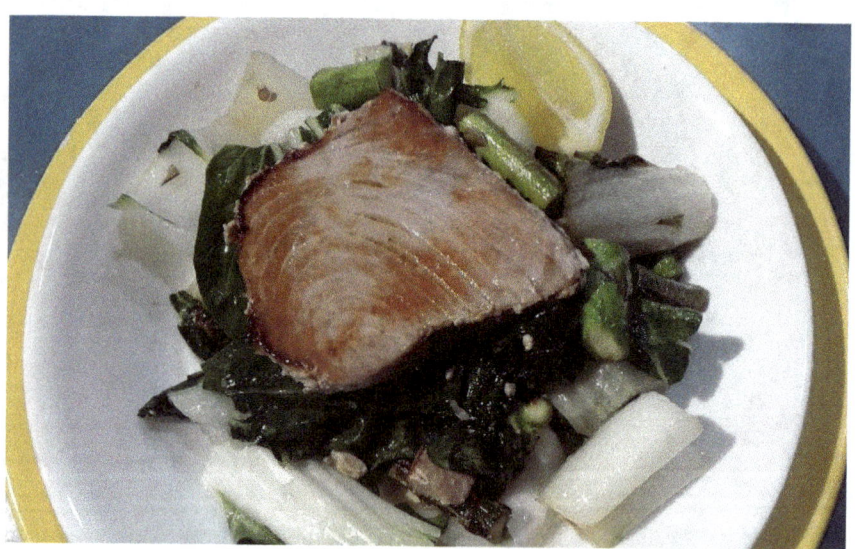

33. Pan-fried tuna bowl, greens, lemon

- Pan-fry tuna steak in olive oil, salt
- Add chopped broccolini, bok choy
- Add juice of one lemon
  In serving bowl
- Add cup of crunchy coleslaw
- Dollop of Greek yoghurt
- Sprinkling of fresh red chili
- Add sliced tuna and cooked vegetables
- Season to taste

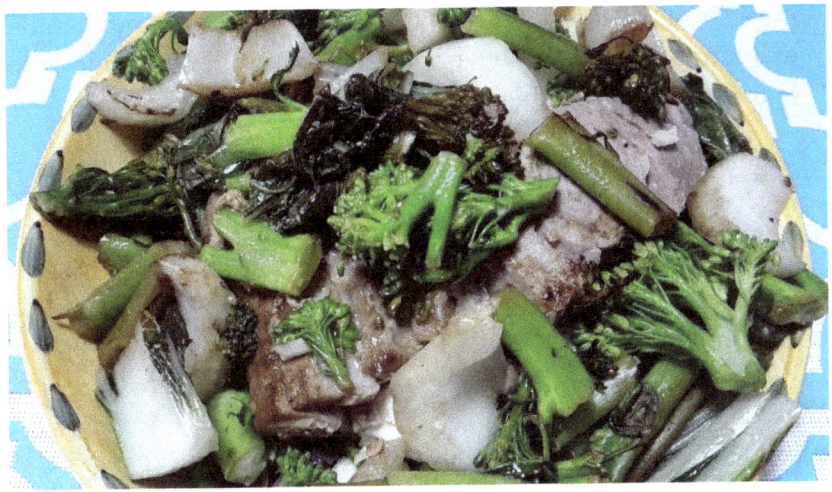

34. Pan-fried tuna bowl, broccoli

- Pan-fry tuna steak in olive oil, salt, pepper
- Add chopped broccoli
  In serving bowl
- Add cup of mixed coleslaw
- Dollop of Greek yoghurt
- ¼ avocado
- Sprinkling of fresh red chili
- Add sliced tuna and cooked broccoli
- Drizzle with Vietnamese Dipping Sauce

Many of these dishes look alike, but you can see how even the most subtle differences can change the look and flavour profile of a familiar recipe. Use what you have in the fridge, and give leftover salad vegetables another life.

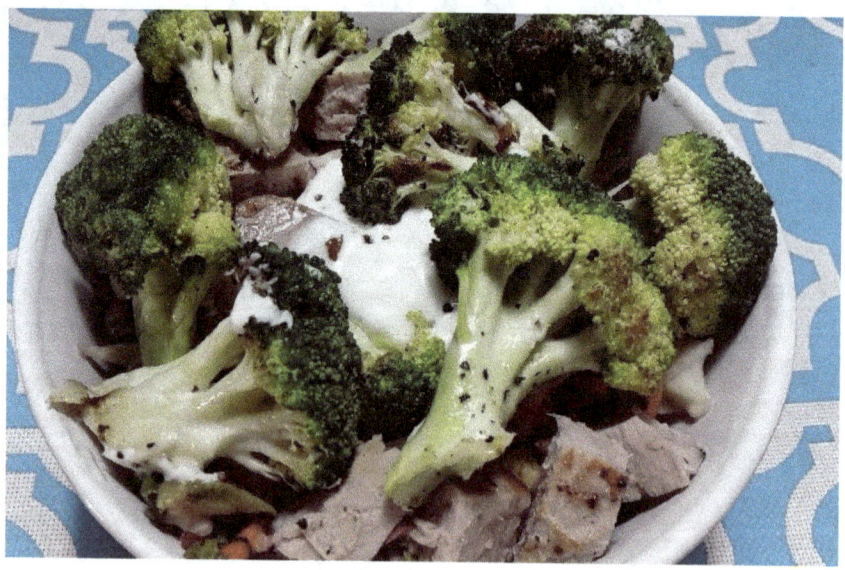

35. Garlic tuna bowl, Pad Thai stir-fry

- Pan-fry tuna in olive oil, with teaspoon each of sambal oelek, chopped garlic, Pad Thai Paste
- Add chopped broccoli, silverbeet, broccolini, coleslaw
- When cooked, take off the heat and slice tuna
- Transfer cooked vegetables to a serving bowl
- Top with sliced tuna, lime wedges
- Drizzle with Obento Sushi & Sashimi Light Soy Sauce

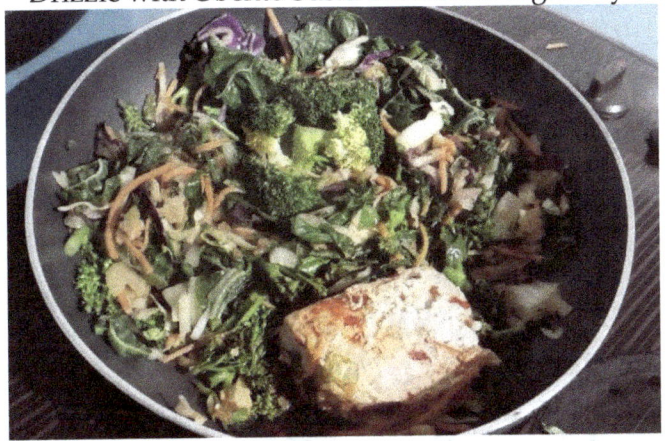

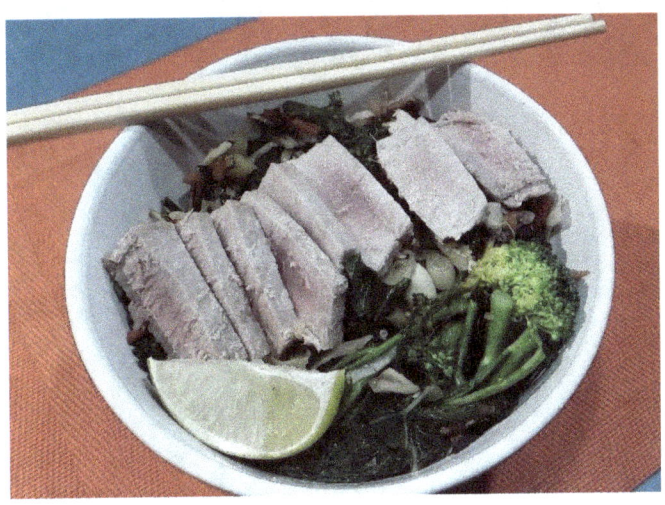

36. Pan-fried tuna bowl, tomato, olives

- Dry pan-fry tuna steak in hot pan (without oil)
- Add chopped silverbeet, Roma tomato
- Add ½ pack of Asian Stir-fry Salad veges
- Add grated fennel bulb and a few black olives
- Add a little oil and cracked pepper, but no salt
- When cooked, take off the heat and slice tuna
- Transfer cooked vegetables to a serving bowl
- Top with sliced tuna, Thai basil
- Drizzle with Chang's Crispy Noodle Salad Dressing (for a touch of toasted sesame)

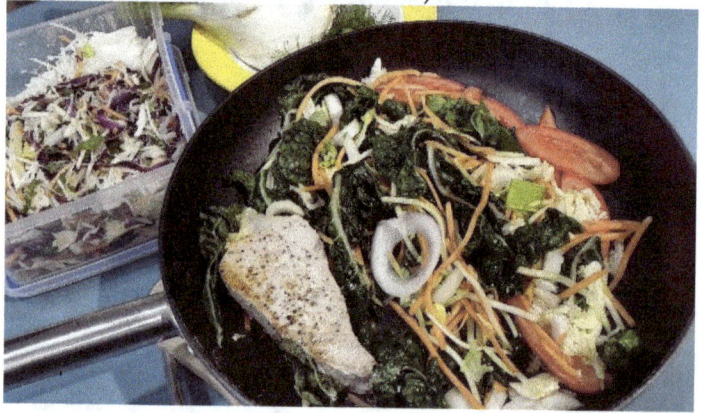

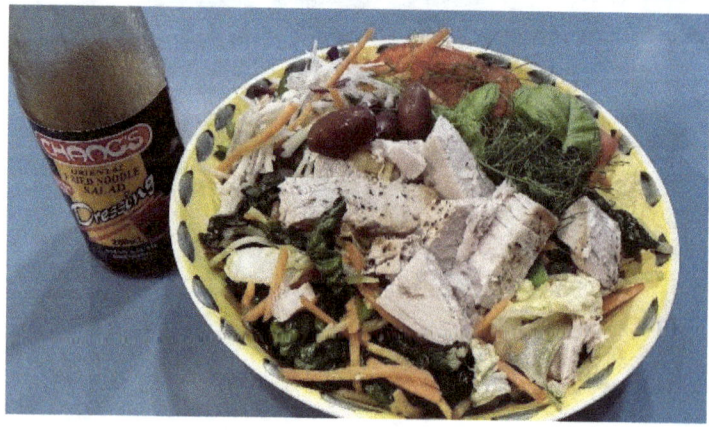

37. Pan-fried tuna bowl, sweet potato, veg

- Pan-fry tuna steak in olive oil
- Add grated sweet potato, salt, cracked pepper
- Add bok choy
- Add cup of mixed coleslaw salad vegetables
- When cooked, transfer everything to a serving bowl
- Drizzle with Japanese Tonkatsu Sauce

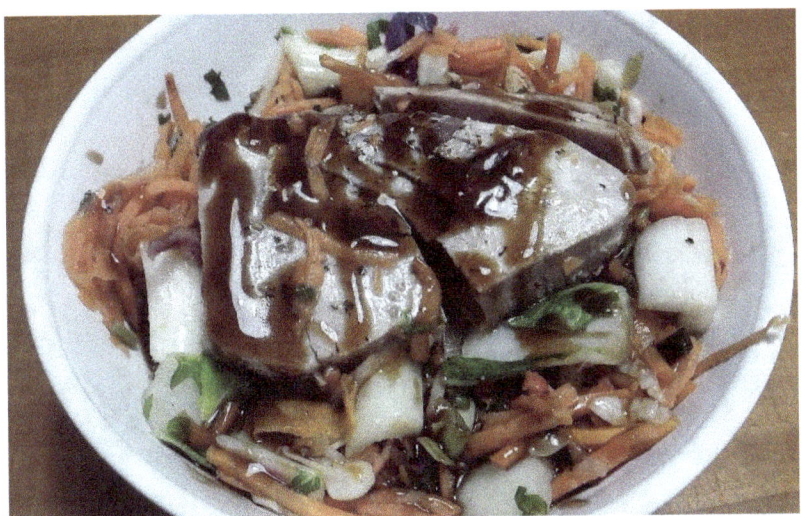

38. Pan-fried tuna bowl, veg, avocado

- Pan-fry tuna steak in olive oil, salt pepper
- Add chopped chili, shallot, broccoli
  Serving
- Add cup of mixed coleslaw salad to a bowl
- Drizzle with coleslaw dressing
- Add ¼ avocado
- Add sliced jalapenos
- Add Vietnamese mint
- Add cooked vegetables on top
- Finish with slices of cooked tuna and lime juice

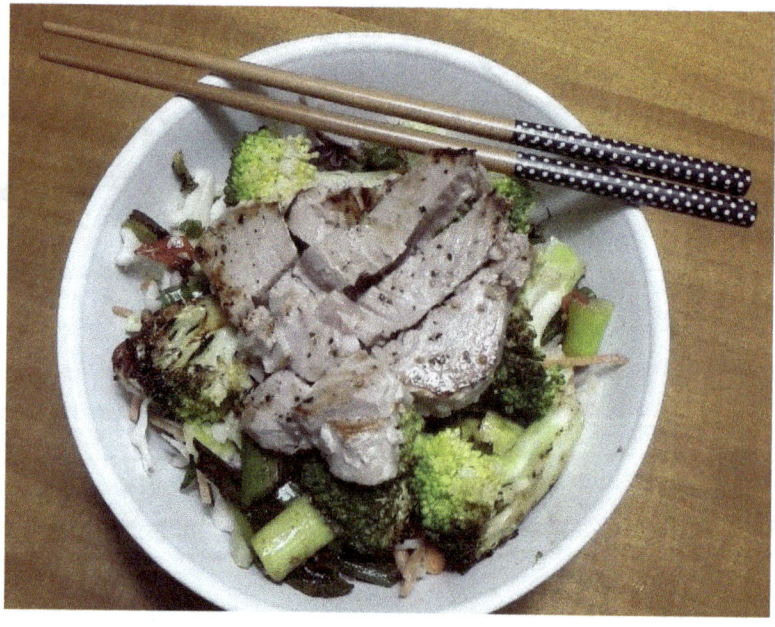

39. Pan-fried tuna, mushrooms, greens

- Add olive oil to hot pan
- Add sliced mushrooms, salt, cracked pepper, then stir
- Add tuna steak
- Add chopped broccoli, silverbeet
- Add cup of mixed coleslaw salad vegetables
- When cooked, slice tuna and transfer everything to a serving bowl
- Serve with squeeze of lime juice.

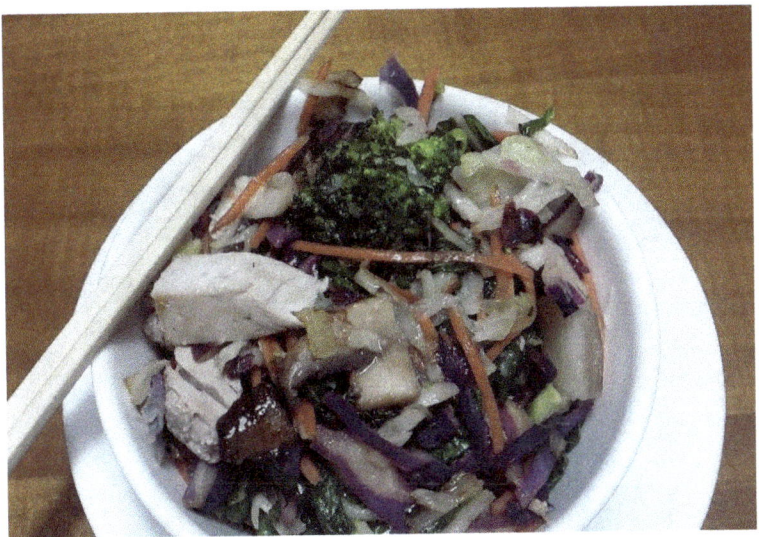

40. Pan-fried tuna, asparagus, noodle salad

- Reconstitute a serve of vermicelli rice noodles. Drain and set aside.
- Add olive oil to hot frying pan, with salt, pepper
- Pan-fry tuna steak and asparagus
  In a serving bowl,
- Add cooked noodles
- Add cup of mixed coleslaw/kaleslaw, alfalfa sprouts
- Add tomato wedges, chopped chili, sliced jalapenos
- Add sliced cooked tuna and asparagus
- Drizzle with Vietnamese dipping sauce
- Add herbs (Thai basil, Viet mint, fennel)
- A spoonful of cottage cheese is optional.

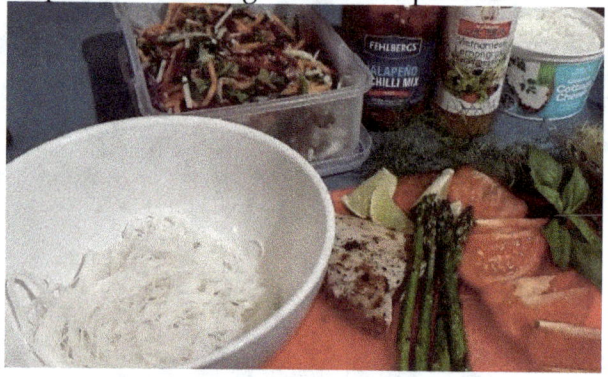

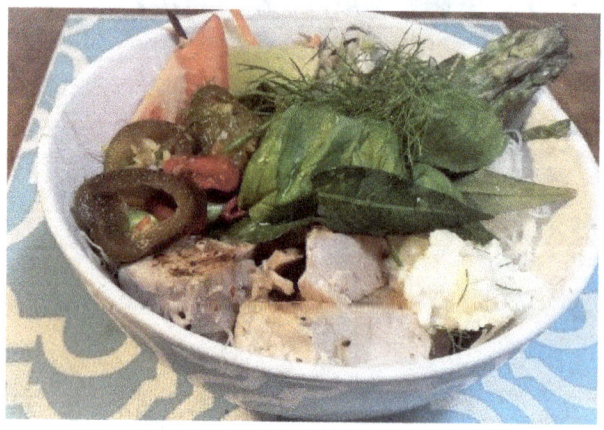

41. Pan-fried tuna, balsamic, noodle salad

- Reconstitute a serve of vermicelli rice noodles. Drain and set aside.
- To a hot pan, add olive oil, sesame oil, balsamic vinegar
- Add thawed tuna steak
- Pan-fry tuna on both sides, season with salt and pepper
- When cooked, remove from heat and slice.

In a serving bowl,

- Add cup of mixed coleslaw salad (dry)
- Add shredded lettuce
- Add cooked vermicelli noodles
- Add diced fresh tomato
- Add sliced cooked tuna
- Add pickled pink sushi ginger
- Add sliced jalapenos
- Drizzle with Balsamic vinegar over tomatoes
- Drizzle Vietnamese dipping sauce over tuna

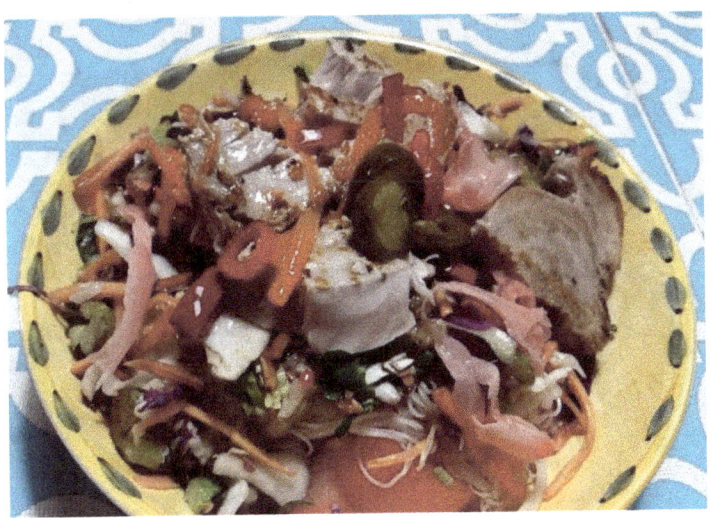

42. Pan-fried tuna, silverbeet, noodle salad

- Reconstitute a serve of vermicelli rice noodles. Drain and set aside.
- To a hot pan, add olive oil, sesame oil, balsamic vinegar
- Add chopped silverbeet
- Add thawed tuna steak. Season with salt, pepper
- Pan-fry tuna on both sides. When cooked, remove pan from heat and slice tuna.
  In a serving bowl,
- Add cup of mixed coleslaw/kaleslaw salad (dry)
- Add cooked vermicelli noodles
- Add sliced cooked tuna
- Add pickled pink sushi ginger
- Add sliced jalapenos
- Drizzle Vietnamese dipping sauce over everything

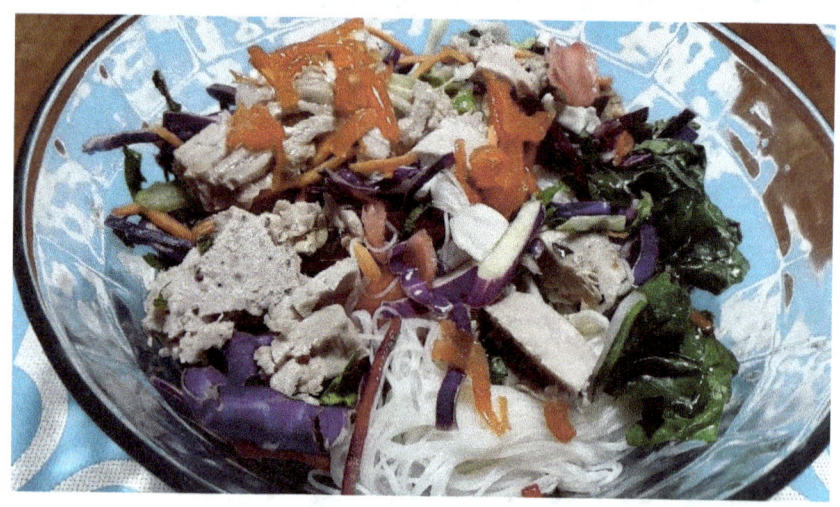

43. Pan-fried tuna, chilled noodle salad

- Reconstitute a serve of vermicelli rice noodles. Drain and set aside.
- Pan-fry thawed tuna steak in hot pan, with salt, pepper
- When browned on both sides, and pink in the middle, remove from heat and slice tuna.
  In a serving bowl,
- Add cooked vermicelli noodles, chilled
- Add cup of mixed coleslaw and mizuna salad (dry)
- Add sliced fresh tomato
- Add sliced cooked tuna
- Drizzle with Chang's Crispy Noodle dressing and a little Vietnamese dipping sauce
- Finish with chopped coriander. Season to taste.

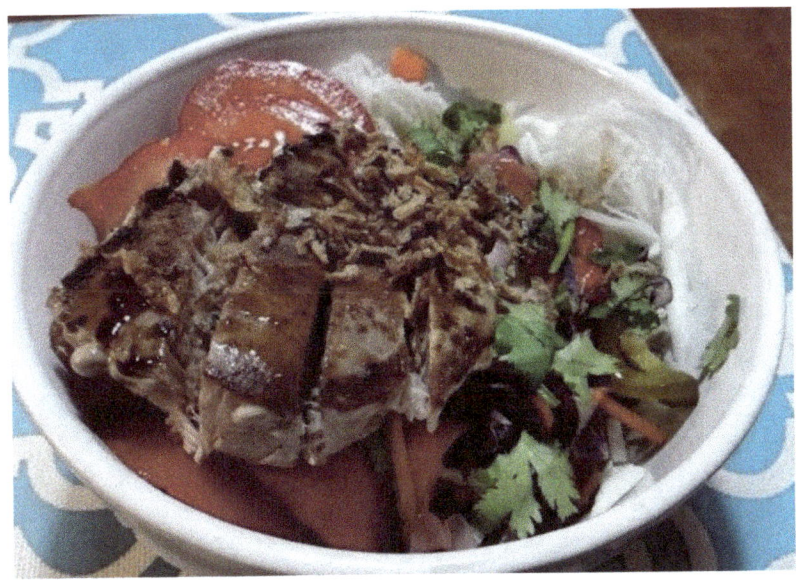

44. Pan-fried tuna, pineapple, noodle salad

- Reconstitute a serve of vermicelli rice noodles. Drain and set aside.
- To a hot pan, add olive oil, cracked pepper
- Add chopped green chili
- Add sliced pineapple and broccolini
- Add thawed tuna steak and pan-fry on both sides
- Remove tuna and slice.

In a serving bowl,
- Add cup of mixed coleslaw/kaleslaw salad (dry)
- Add cooked vermicelli noodles
- Add ½ sliced tomato
- Add pickled pink sushi ginger
- Add alfalfa sprouts
- Add sliced cooked tuna
- Add cooked broccolini and pineapple
- Finish with Vietnamese mint, a drizzle of Vietnamese Lemongrass Dressing, and a dollop of Greek yoghurt

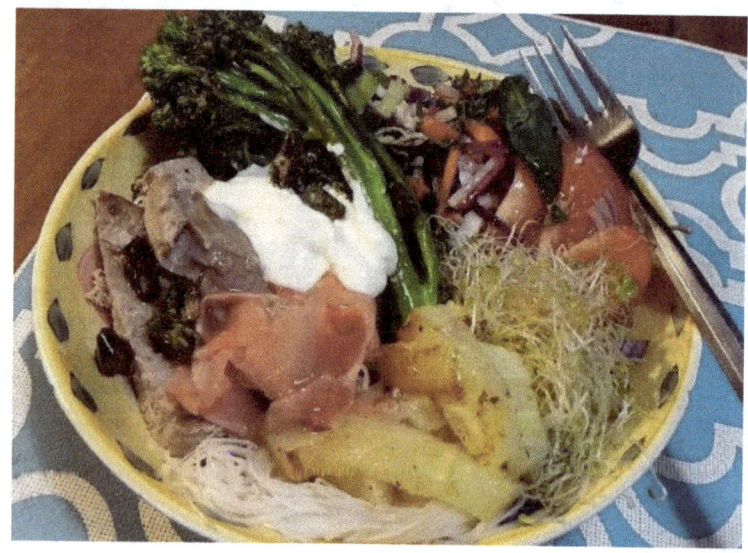

45. Pan-fried tuna, stir-fried veg, noodles

- Reconstitute a serve of vermicelli rice noodles. Drain and set aside.
- To a hot pan, add olive oil, cracked pepper
- Stir-fry pineapple, broccolini, mushrooms, silverbeet, asparagus
- Add thawed tuna steak and pan-fry on both sides
- Remove tuna and slice.

  In a serving bowl,
- Add cooked vermicelli noodles
- Add cooked vegetables and sliced tuna
- Add ¼ avocado
- Add pickled pink sushi ginger
- Add sliced pickled jalapenos and chilis
- Finish with Vietnamese mint, and lemon juice

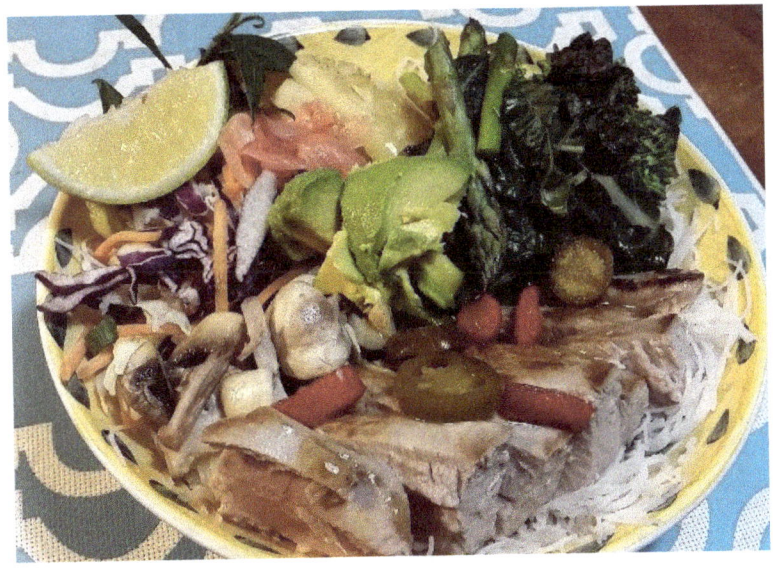

46. Pan-fried tuna, hoisin veg, flat noodles

- In a saucepan, cook 50g of flat rice noodles in boiling water for about 6 minutes. Drain and set aside.
- In a hot frying pan, add olive oil, sambal oelek chili paste, and cracked pepper
- Add thawed tuna steak (pan-fry on both sides)
- Stir-fry chopped wombok, choy sum, kaleslaw, with a splash of hoisin and fish sauces
- Remove tuna and slice.
  In a serving bowl,
- Add cooked vermicelli noodles
- Add cooked vegetables and sliced tuna
- Finish with a splash of soy sauce, chopped Asian herbs

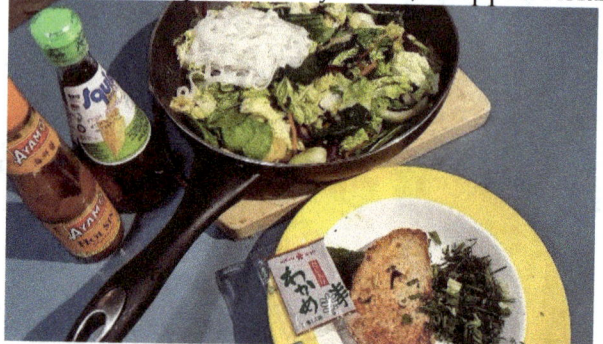

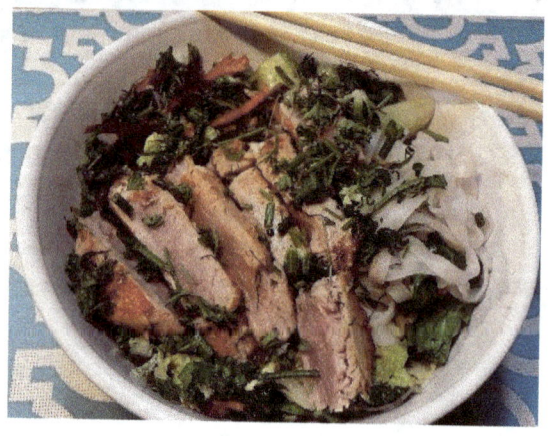

47. Braised tuna, miso, noodles

- Reconstitute a serve of vermicelli rice noodles. Drain and set aside.
- To a hot pan, add olive oil, cracked pepper
- Pan-fry tuna on both sides
- Add broccolini
- Add cup of mixed coleslaw veg
- Add teaspoon of MISO PASTE mixed with a cup of boiling water, or a use sachet of miso soup with water
- Remove tuna and slice.

  In a serving bowl,
- Add cup of mixed coleslaw/kaleslaw salad (dry)
- Add cooked vermicelli noodles
- Add sliced cooked tuna
- Add cooked vegetables and pan juices
- Drizzle with Chang's Crispy Noodle Dressing

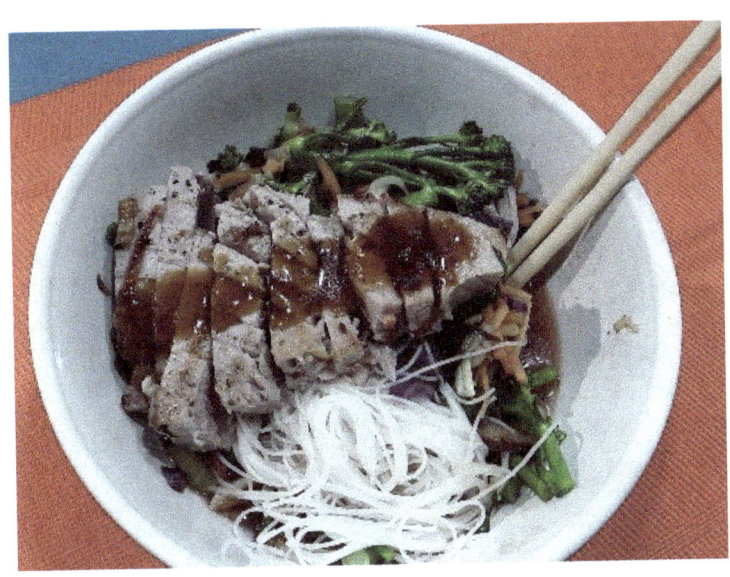

48. Braised tuna Tom Yum, chili, noodles

- Reconstitute a serve of vermicelli rice noodles. Drain and set aside.
- Add olive oil to hot frying pan, with salt, pepper
- Add sliced zucchini, and ½ green chili, chopped
- Add thawed tuna steak (sear one side, then flip to sear other side)
- Add cup of mixed dry coleslaw
- Add tablespoon chopped fresh parsley
- Remove tuna and slice. Return to pan.
- Mix large teaspoon TOM YUM paste with cup of water. Add to pan. Add cooked vermicelli rice noodles.
- Stir to combine. Allow to simmer for a minute.
- Transfer to bowl. Finish with squeeze of lime juice.

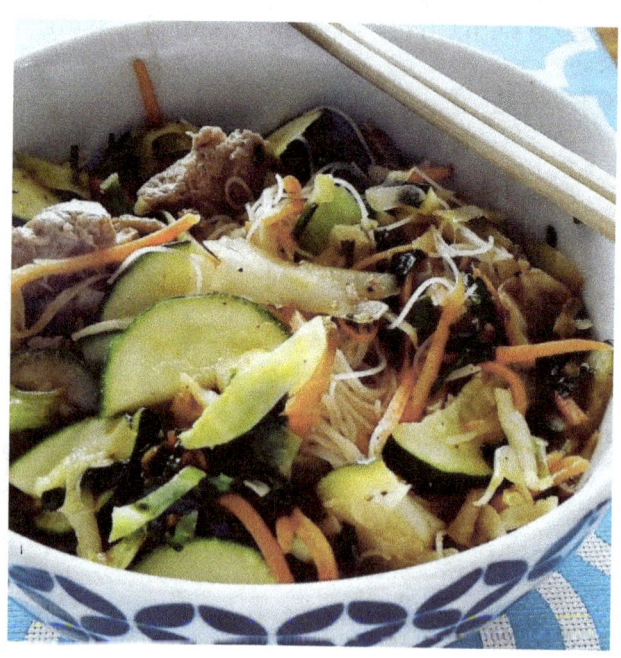

49. Braised tuna, yellow curry noodle soup

- Prepare a serve of flat rice noodles by cooking in a saucepan of boiling water for a few minutes. Drain and set aside.

- Add olive oil to a hot frying pan
- Add sliced mushrooms, salt, cracked pepper, then stir
- Add chopped broccoli, Asian leafy greens (gai lan or choy sum)
- Add cup of mixed coleslaw salad vegetables
- Mix large teaspoon of Yellow Curry Paste (Indian style) with a cup of water. Add to pan and bring to boil.
- Add thin slices of raw tuna (easy to cut thinly when only partially thawed)
- Submerge tuna slices in pan juices, and allow to cook for a minute or two. Then remove pan from heat.
- Serve in a bowl with flat rice noodles
- Top with a squeeze of lime juice and dollop of yoghurt.

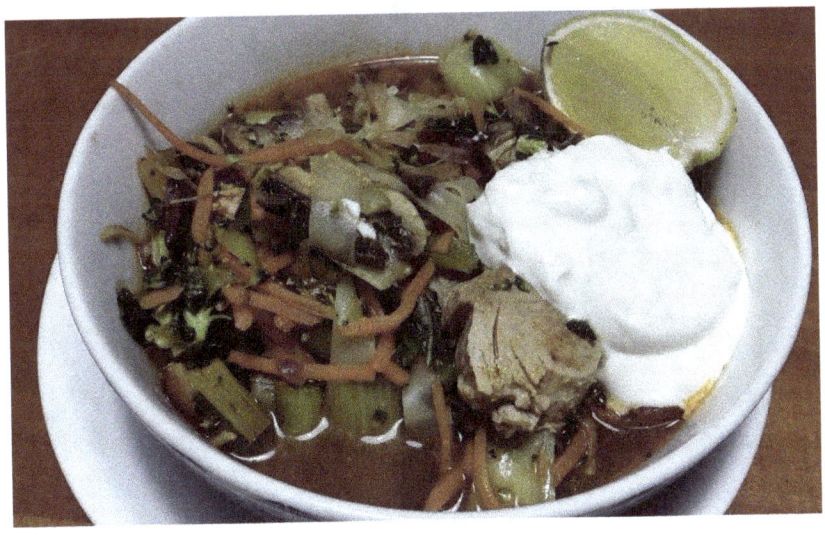

50. Poached Malaysian tuna, flat noodles

- Prepare a serve of flat rice noodles by cooking in a saucepan of boiling water for a few minutes. Drain and set aside.

- Add olive oil to a hot frying pan
- Add sliced mushrooms, salt, cracked pepper, then stir
- Add chopped broccoli, Asian leafy greens (gai lan or choy sum)
- Add cup of mixed coleslaw salad vegetables
- Add splash of fish sauce, and vinegar
- Mix large teaspoon of Malaysian Laksa Paste with a cup of water. Add to pan and bring to boil.
- Add thin slices of raw tuna (easy to cut thinly when only partially thawed). Submerge tuna slices in pan juices, and allow to cook for a minute or two. Then remove pan from heat.
- Serve in a bowl with flat rice noodles
- Finish with a squeeze of lime juice if desired.

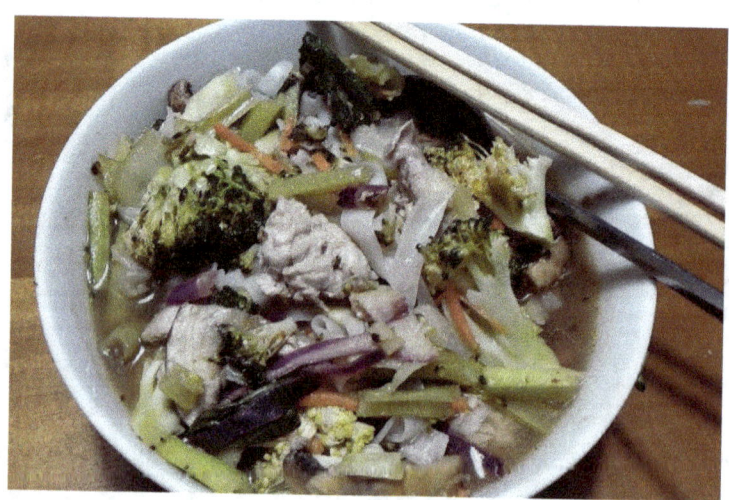

51. Poached miso tuna soup, flat noodles

- Add 2 cups of chicken stock to a saucepan and bring to the boil
- Stir in a large teaspoon of Japanese miso paste (or a sachet of miso soup concentrate)
- Add 50g dried flat ribbon rice noodles and cook for 5 minutes
- Add ½ baby bok choy
- Cut a partially-thawed tuna steak into thin strips and add to the soup
- Remove from heat and transfer to a bowl.
- Serve with Vietnamese-style toppings (coriander, Vietnamese mint, lemon juice, chili).
- Balance flavours with a dash of soy and/or fish sauce.

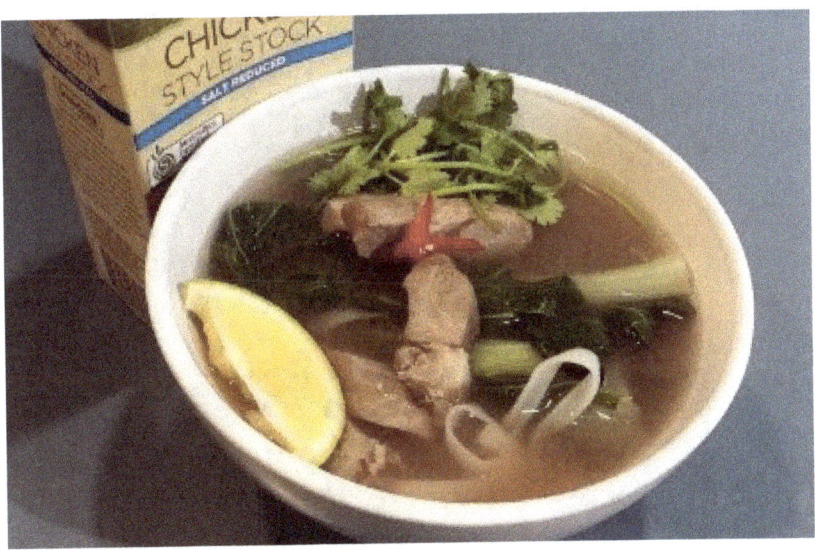

52. Instant pho, tuna, bok choy, flat noodles

- **Lian Pho Bo Vietnamese Style instant rice noodle soup, 70g, with flavour sachets, in a plastic bowl**
- Open the flavour sachets and sprinkle them over the dried vermicelli noodles in the plastic bowl. Then cover with boiling water until about an inch from the rim.
- Loosely cover with lid for a couple of minutes.
- Remove lid and stir softened noodles.
- Cut a partially-thawed tuna steak into thin strips and add to the soup with chopped baby bok choy. Cover for a couple of minutes to keep the heat in.
- Serve with Vietnamese-style toppings (coriander, Vietnamese mint, lemon juice, chili).
- Balance flavours with a dash of soy and/or fish sauce.

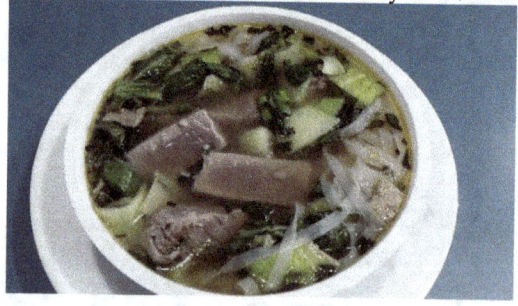

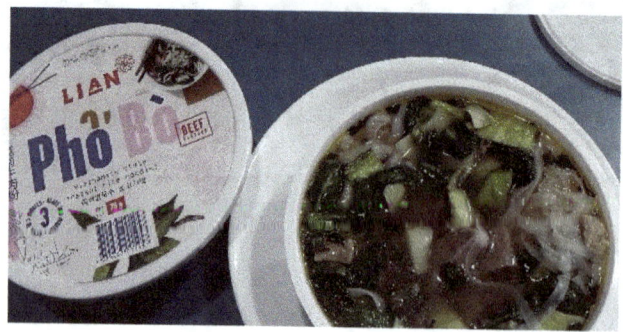

NEW ZEALAND HOKI

Fillets of white fish – such as Hoki, barramundi, whiting, or cod – are easy to cook when you know how, and infinitely versatile as a quality protein source in tasty, low-calorie meals. Mild in flavour, white fish fillets work well in almost any recipe using fish.

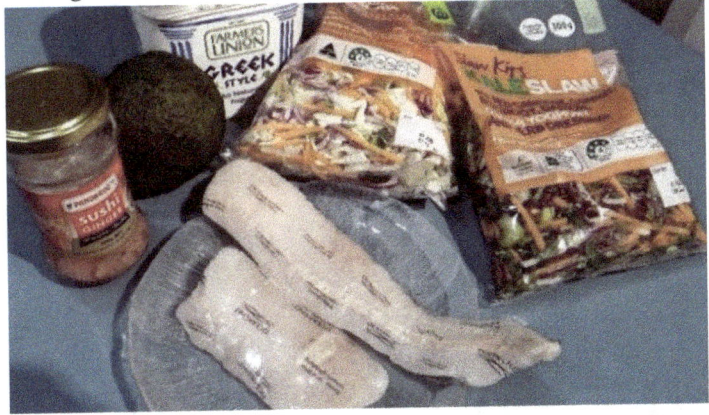

- **Ocean Chef** Hoki Fillets, individually wrapped, 1kg pack (from Woolworths)

These wild-caught Blue Grenadier, also known as Hoki, are caught in the deep waters off New Zealand. Fillets are individually wrapped in plastic, which helps to protect the fish from freezer burn. For these recipes, buy fillets without skin.

53. Hoki rolls, avo, jalapenos

- Hoki fillet pan-fried in olive oil, cracked pepper, salt
- 3 rice paper rounds
- Pickled pink sushi ginger
- ¼ avocado
- Sliced jalapenos
- Cup of mixed coleslaw with dressing

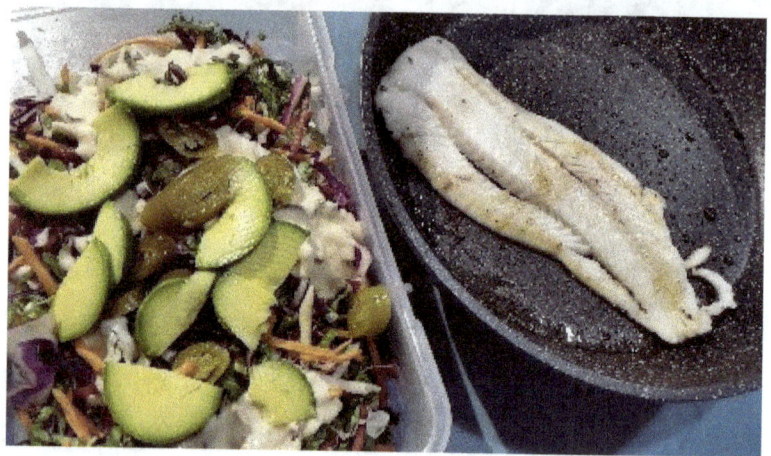

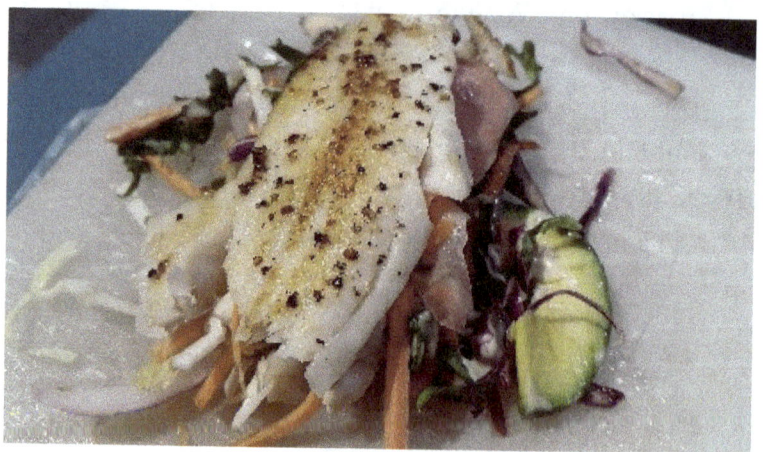

54. Hoki rolls, alfalfa, cos lettuce

- Hoki fillet pan-fried in olive oil, cracked pepper, salt
- 3 rice paper rounds
- Pickled pink sushi ginger
- ¼ avocado
- Sliced jalapenos, and a little vinegar from jar
- Alfalfa sprouts
- Cup of Southern Coleslaw salad kit, with dressing
- Cos lettuce leaves, Vietnamese mint

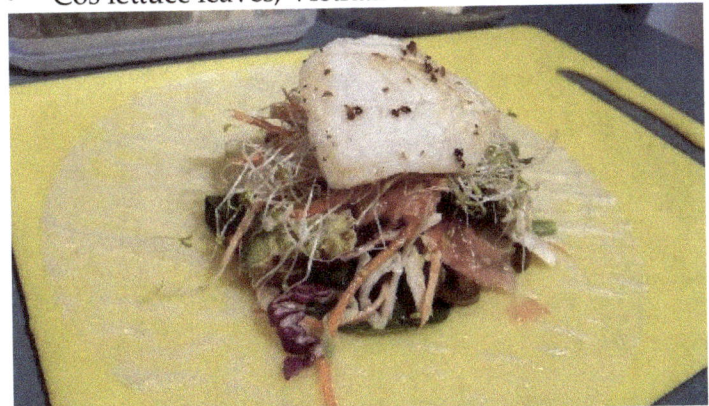

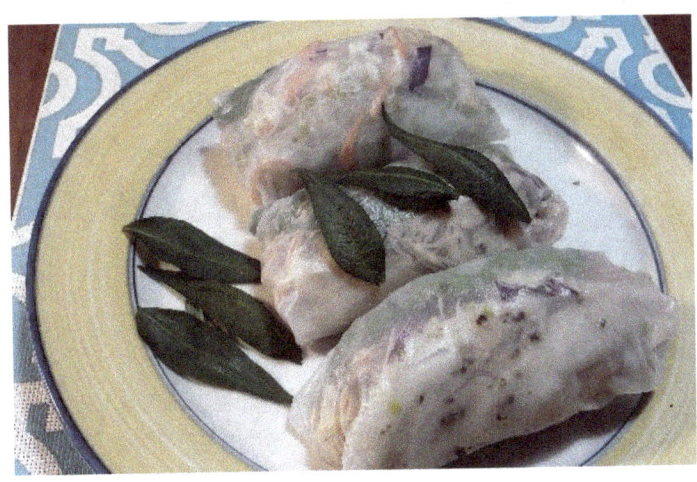

55. Hoki rolls, capers, avo

- Hoki fillet pan-fried in olive oil, capers, salt
- 3 rice paper rounds
- Pickled pink sushi ginger
- ¼ avocado
- Cup of Southern Coleslaw salad kit
- Drizzle of Vietnamese Dipping Sauce

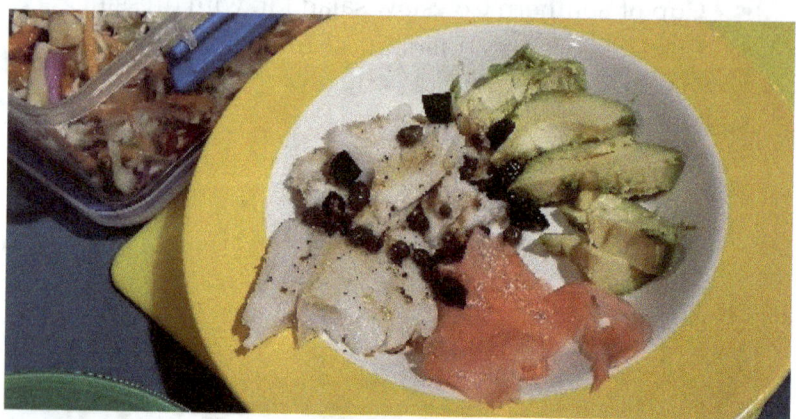

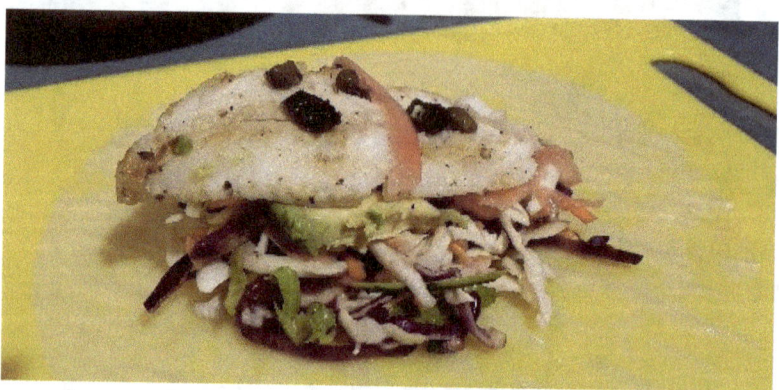

56. Hoki rolls, capers, sambal oelek

- Hoki fillet pan-fried in olive oil, capers, salt
- 3 rice paper rounds
- ¼ avocado
- Greek yoghurt
- Teaspoon sambal oelek chili paste
- Cup of Crunchy Coleslaw salad kit (dry)
- Baby salad leaves
- Thai basil

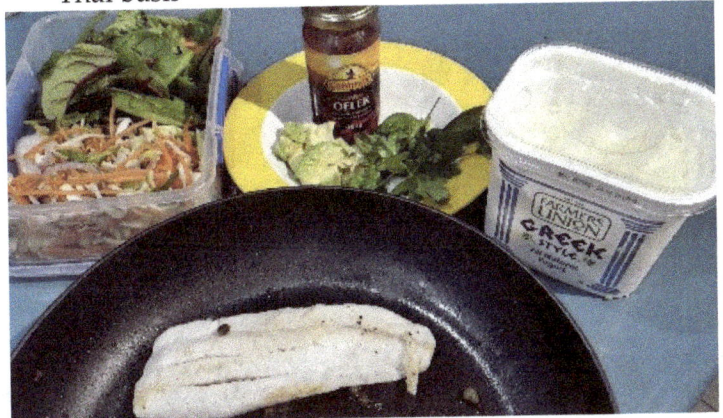

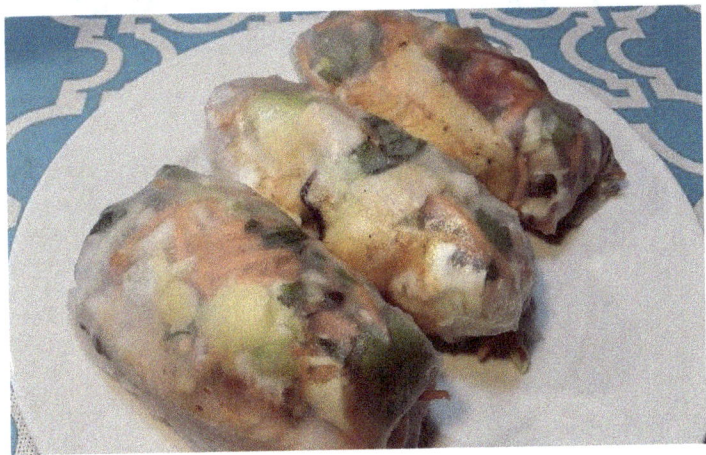

57. Hoki rolls, garlic, chili

- Hoki fillets pan-fried in olive oil, garlic, salt
- 3 rice paper rounds
- Pickled pink sushi ginger
- ¼ avocado
- Teaspoon of sambal oelek chili paste
- Alfalfa sprouts, sliced red onion rings
- Cup of mixed coleslaw/kaleslaw (dry)
- Iceberg lettuce leaves, Thai basil, lime juice

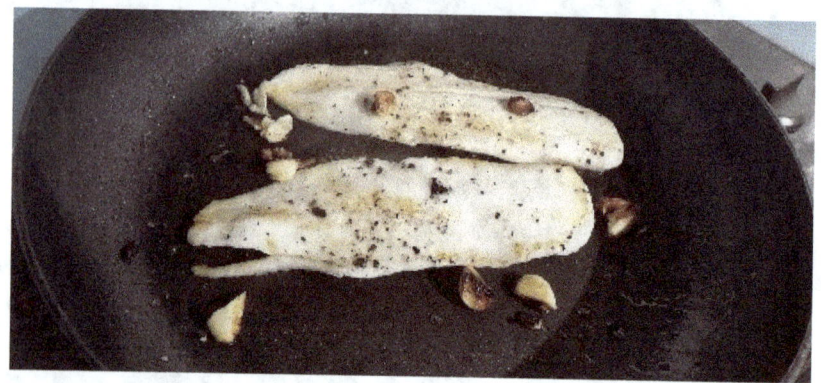

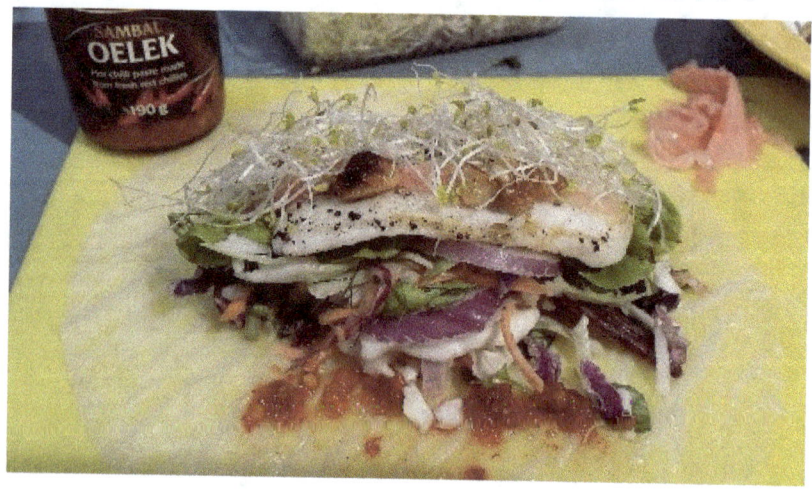

58. Hoki rolls, beetroot, cottage cheese

- Hoki fillets pan-fried in olive oil, onion, chili, salt, cracked pepper
- 3 rice paper rounds
- ¼ avocado
- Sliced tinned beetroot
- Creamed cottage cheese
- Cup of mixed coleslaw/kaleslaw (dry)
- Thai basil, parsley

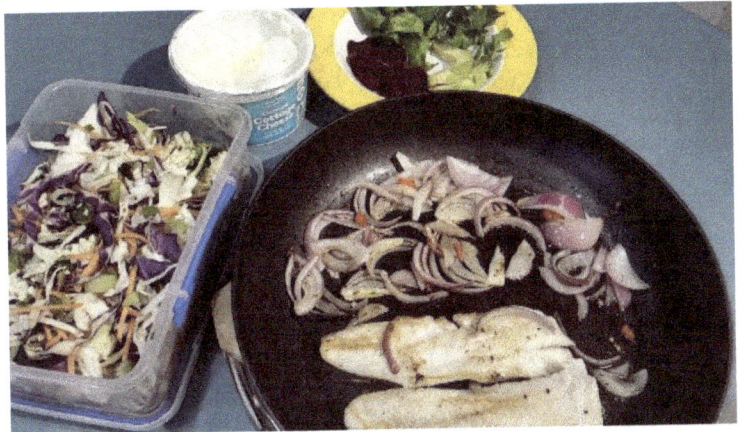

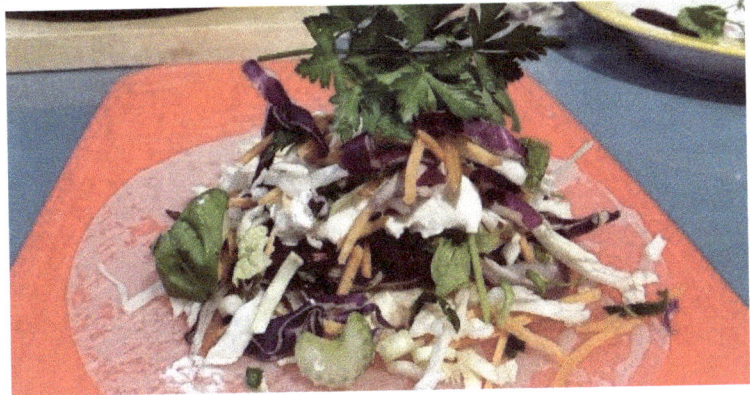

59. Hoki rolls, avo, onion, lime

- Hoki fillets pan-fried in olive oil, salt, cracked pepper
- 3 rice paper rounds
- ¼ avocado, lime juice
- Pickled pink sushi ginger
- Cup of mixed coleslaw, with onion rings and dressing

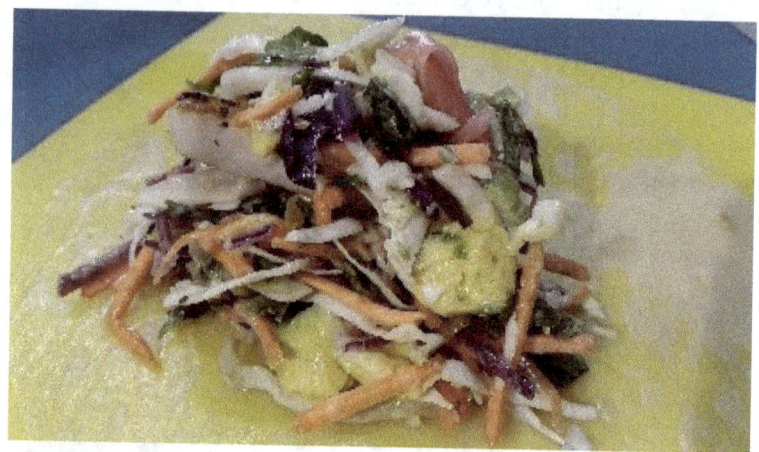

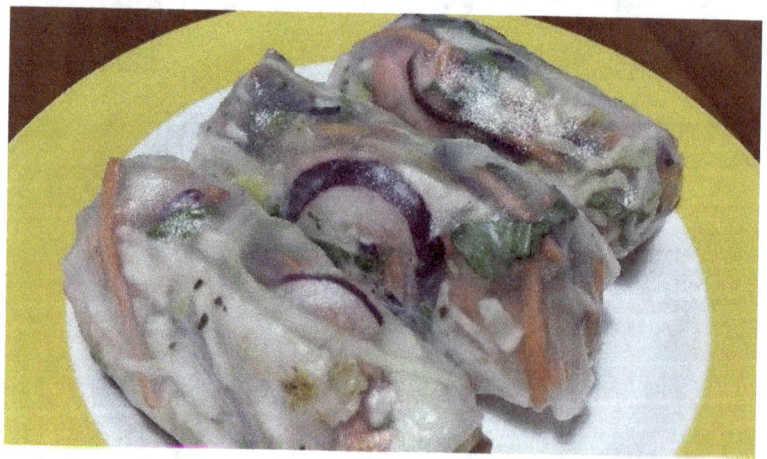

60. Hoki rolls, avo, yoghurt

- Hoki fillets pan-fried in olive oil, salt, cracked pepper
- 3 rice paper rounds
- Jalapenos, and a little vinegar from jar
- ¼ avocado
- Greek yoghurt
- Parsley
- Cup of mixed coleslaw (dry)

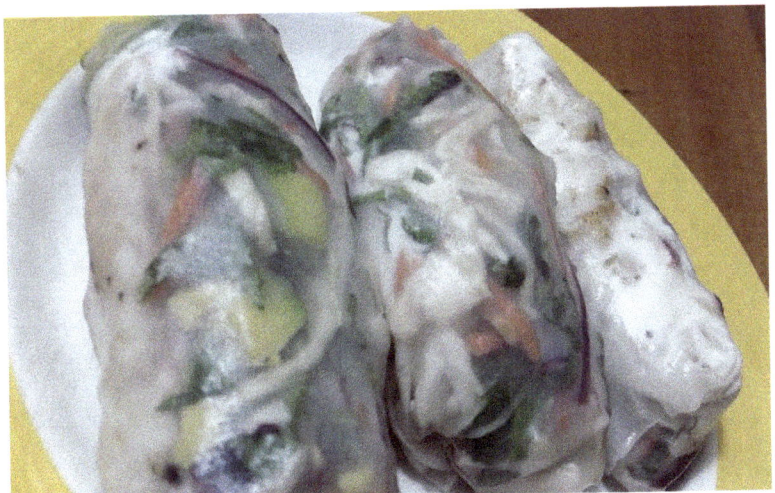

61. Hoki rolls, avo, coleslaw

- Hoki fillets pan-fried in olive oil, salt, cracked pepper
- 3 rice paper rounds
- Pickled pink sushi ginger
- Jalapenos
- ¼ avocado
- Alfalfa sprouts
- Cup of Thai Mizuna Salad mix (dry)
- Thai basil, Vietnamese mint, parsley
- Drizzle with a salad dressing of your choice

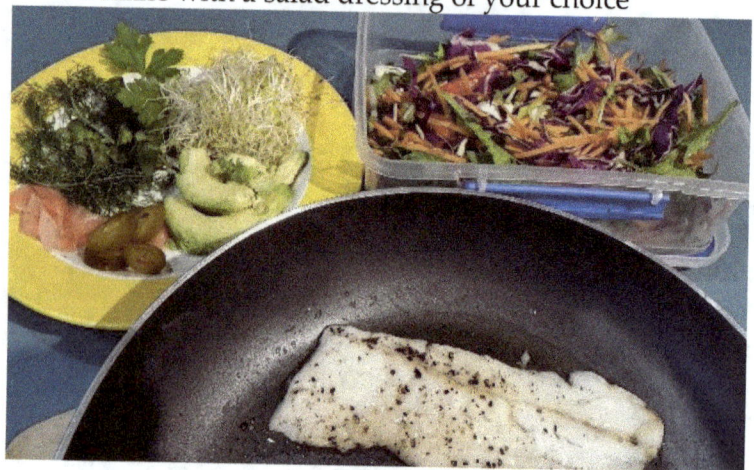

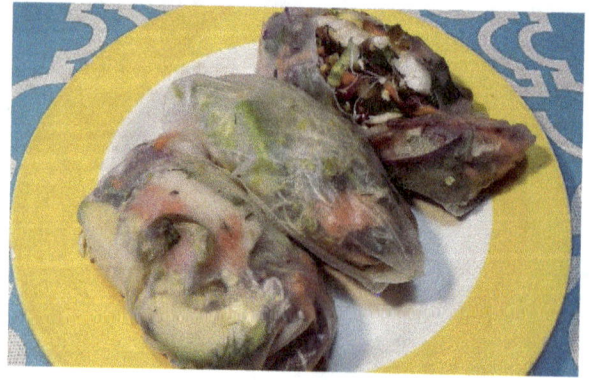

62. Hoki rolls, chili, crispy onion sprinkles

- 2 Hoki fillets pan-fried in olive oil, chili, salt, pepper
- 3 rice paper rounds
- Pickled pink sushi ginger
- ¼ avocado
- Greek yoghurt
- Cup of mixed coleslaw/kaleslaw (dry)
- Finish with sprinkling of crispy fried onion bits that come in a small packet with some of the salad kits

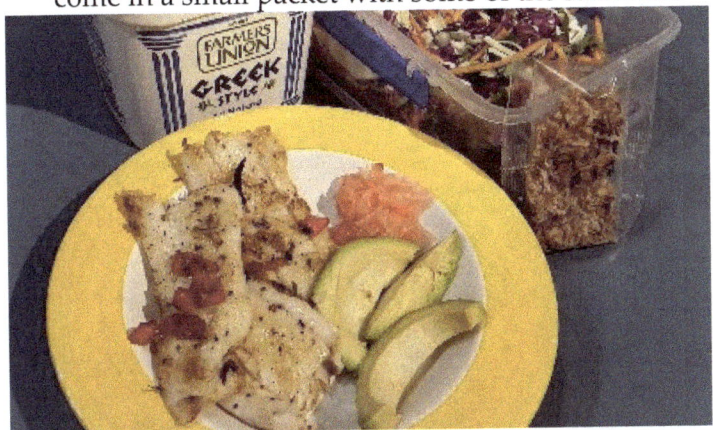

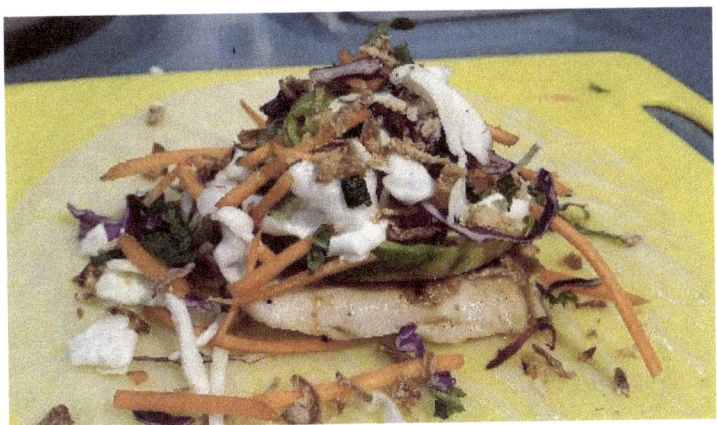

63. Hoki rolls, nori, cos lettuce

- Hoki fillet pan-fried in olive oil, cracked pepper, salt
- 3 rice paper rounds
- Pickled pink sushi ginger
- ¼ avocado
- Sliced jalapenos, and a little vinegar from jar
- ½ sliced sheet of nori seaweed
- Cup of Southern Coleslaw salad kit, with dressing
- Cos lettuce leaves

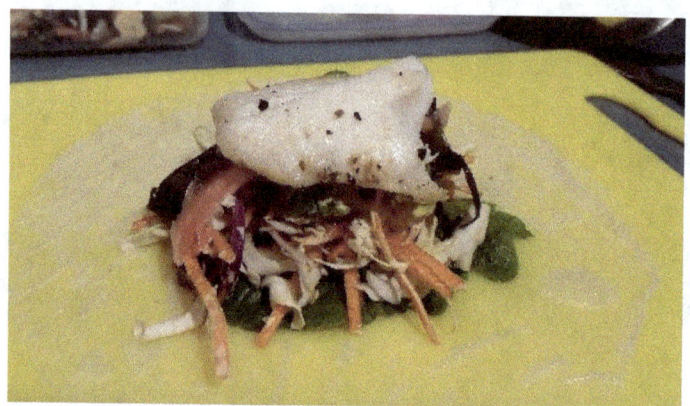

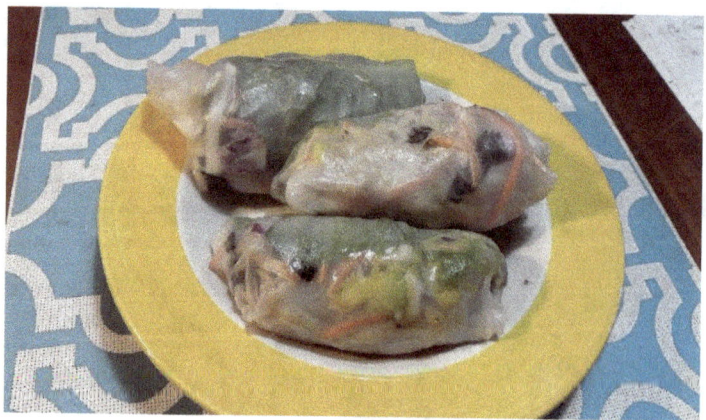

64. Hoki rolls, garlic, chili, nori

- Hoki fillet pan-fried in olive oil, garlic, pickled red chili, cracked pepper, salt
- 3 rice paper rounds
- Pickled pink sushi ginger
- ¼ avocado
- ½ sliced sheet of nori seaweed
- Cup of coleslaw, with dressing
- Butter lettuce

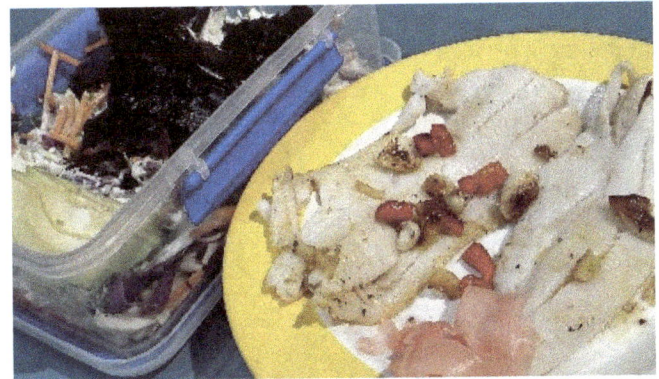

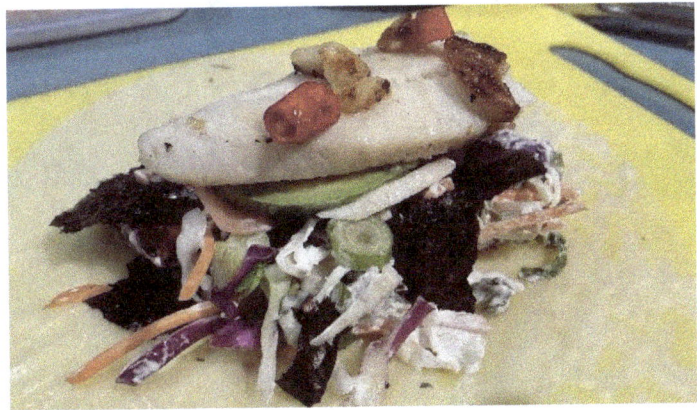

65. Hoki rolls, onion, nori, herbs

- Hoki fillet pan-fried in olive oil, onion, red chili, salt
- 3 rice paper rounds
- Pickled pink sushi ginger
- ¼ avocado
- Greek yoghurt
- ½ sheet nori seaweed, sliced
- Alfalfa sprouts
- Cup of mixed coleslaw/kaleslaw (dry)
- Fennel herb, coriander, Thai basil

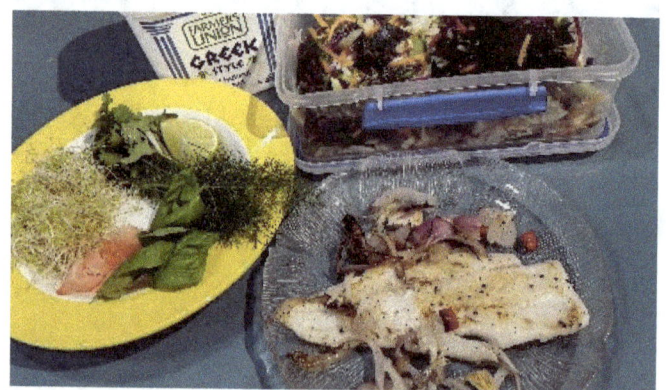

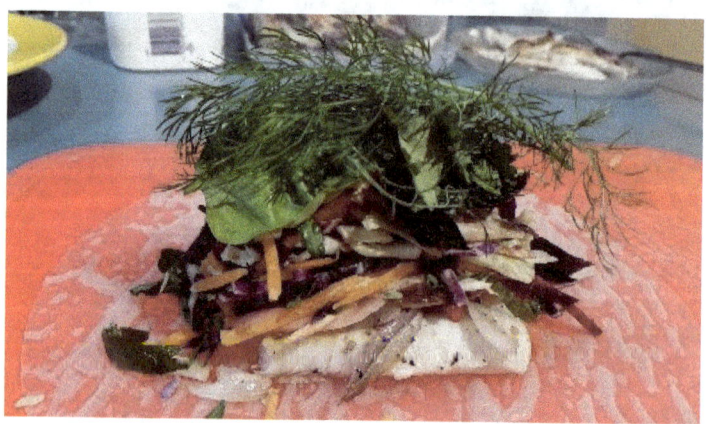

66. Hoki rolls, nori, wasabi, kale

- Dry-fried Hoki fillets in hot pan, salt, pepper
- 3 rice paper rounds
- Pickled pink sushi ginger
- ½ sliced sheet of nori seaweed
- Cup of kaleslaw, with dressing
- Touch of wasabi paste
- Squeeze of lemon juice

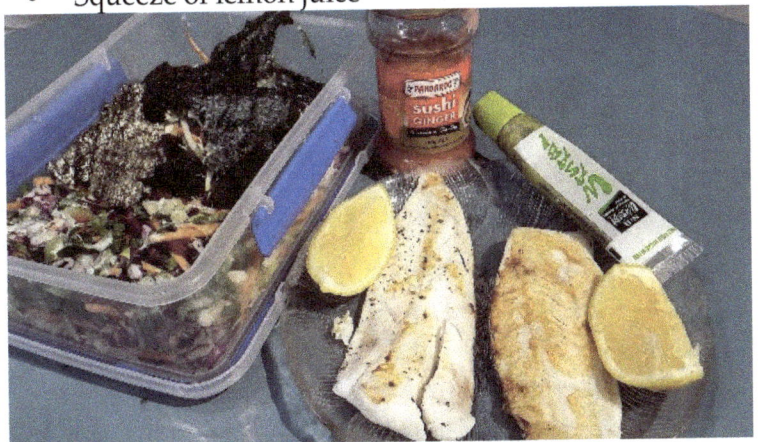

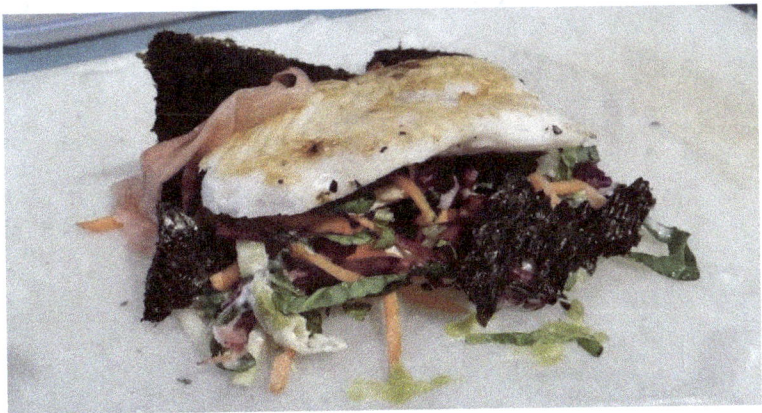

67. Hoki rolls, chili, Mizuna salad

- Hoki fillet pan-fried in olive oil, fresh red chili, cracked pepper, salt
- 3 rice paper rounds
- Pickled pink sushi ginger
- ¼ avocado
- Greek yoghurt
- ½ sliced sheet of nori seaweed
- Cup of mixed coleslaw and Thai Mizuna salad

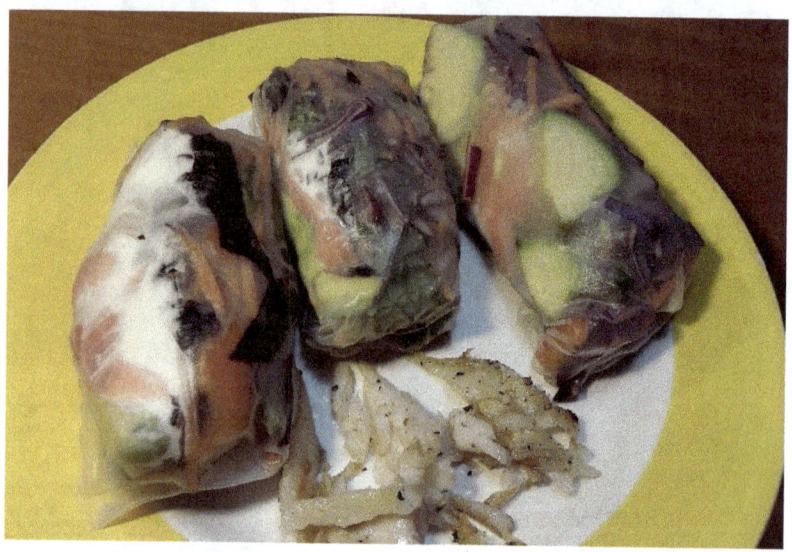

68. Hoki rolls, fried red capsicum, nori

- 2 Hoki fillet pan-fried in olive oil, cracked pepper, salt, thin strips of red capsicum, a teaspoon chopped red chili
- 3 rice paper rounds
- Pickled pink sushi ginger
- ¼ avocado
- Greek yoghurt
- ½ sliced sheet of nori seaweed
- Cup of mixed coleslaw/kaleslaw (dry)
- Coriander

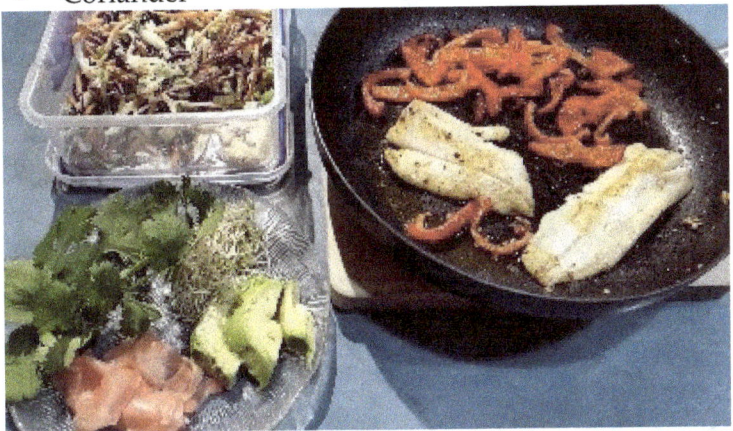

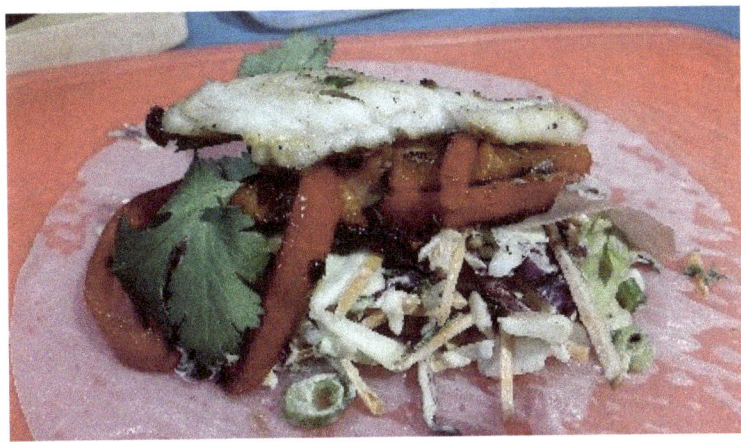

69. Hoki rolls, fried onion, cottage cheese

- 2 Hoki fillet pan-fried in olive oil, cracked pepper, salt, a sliced red onion, a teaspoon chopped red chili
- Stir-fry baby bok choy in same pan.
  Use 3 rice paper rounds to make rolls
- ¼ avocado
- Cottage cheese
- ½ sliced sheet of nori seaweed
- Cup of mixed coleslaw/kaleslaw (dry)
- Coriander
- Serve fried onions and bok choy on the side.

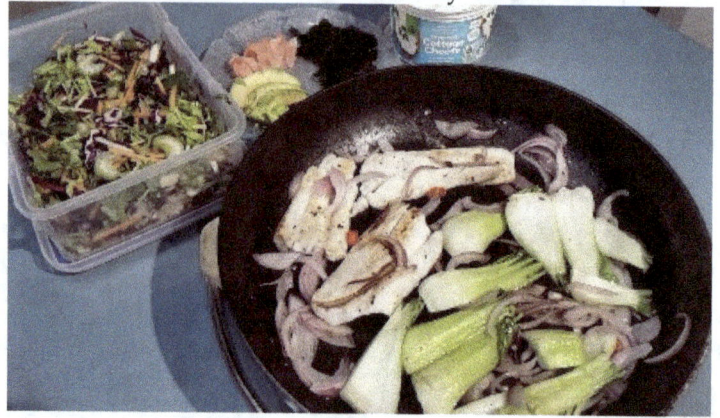

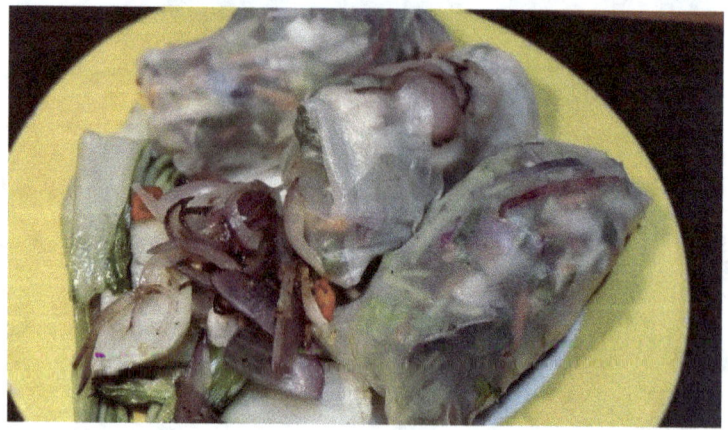

70. Hoki rolls, fried onion, bok choy, chili

- Pan-fry 1-2 Hoki fillets in hot pan, with olive oil, cracked pepper, salt, a sliced red onion, garlic, chili
- Stir-fry baby bok choy in same pan.
  Use 3 rice paper rounds to make rolls:
- Pickled pink sushi ginger
- ¼ avocado, lime juice
- Greek yoghurt
- Alfalfa, Thai basil, fennel herb
- Cup of mixed coleslaw/kaleslaw (dry)

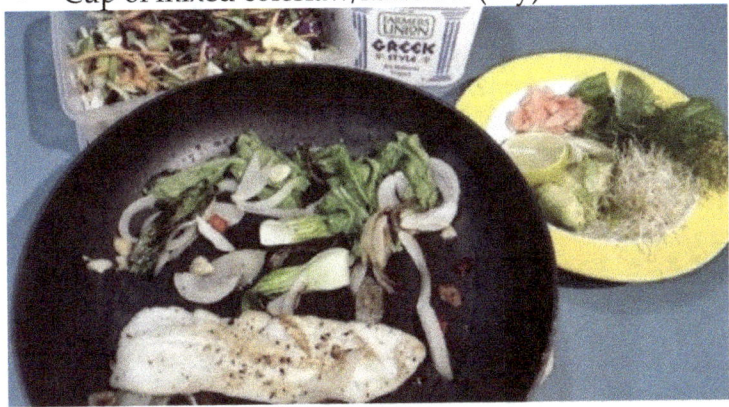

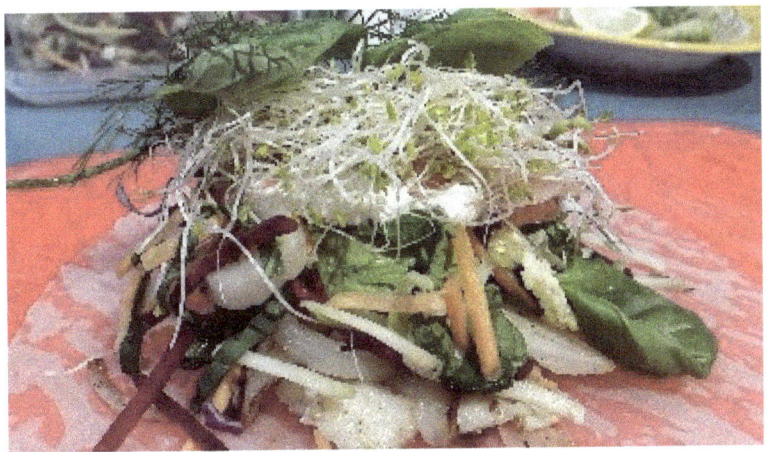

71. Hoki rolls, broccolini, avo

- Hoki fillet pan-fried in olive oil, cracked pepper, salt
- Pan-fry broccolini in same pan
  Use 3 rice paper rounds to make rolls
- Pickled pink sushi ginger
- Jalapenos
- ¼ avocado
- Alfalfa sprouts
- Cup of mixed coleslaw/kaleslaw, with dressing
- Serve broccolini on the side.

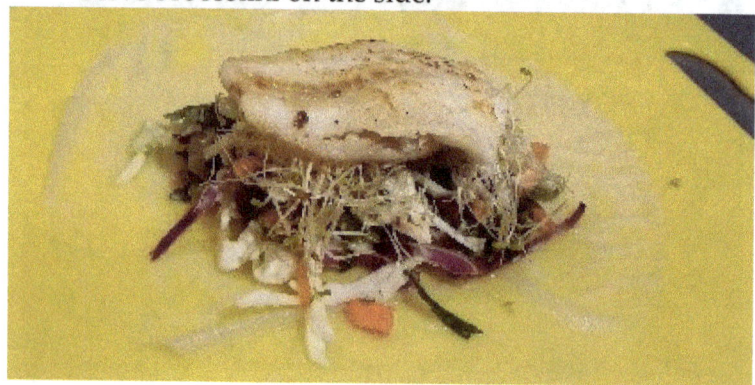

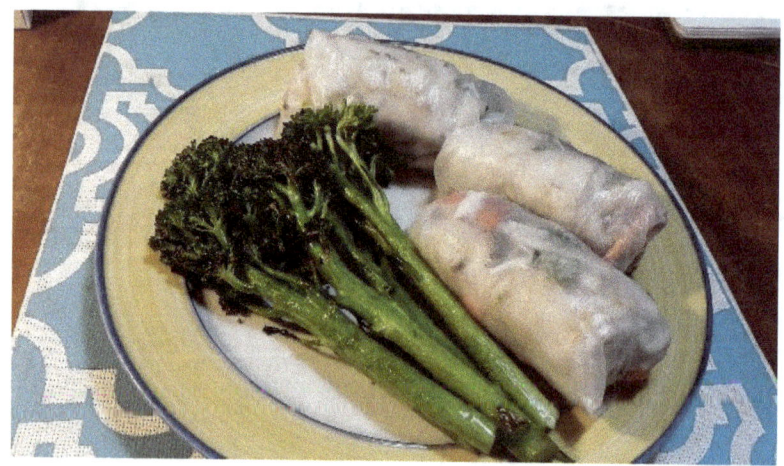

72. Hoki rolls, pineapple, broccolini

- Hoki fillet pan-fried in olive oil, cracked pepper, salt, garlic, red chili
- Add sliced pineapple, broccolini, bok choy to pan
  Use 3 rice paper rounds to make rolls
- Pickled pink sushi ginger
- Cup of mixed coleslaw/kaleslaw
- Dill, fennel herb, Green Seafood Dipping Sauce
- Serve Hoki salad rolls with fried veges on the side.

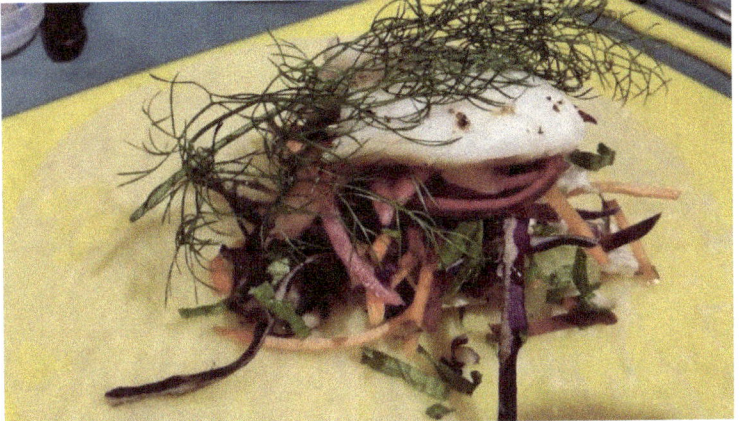

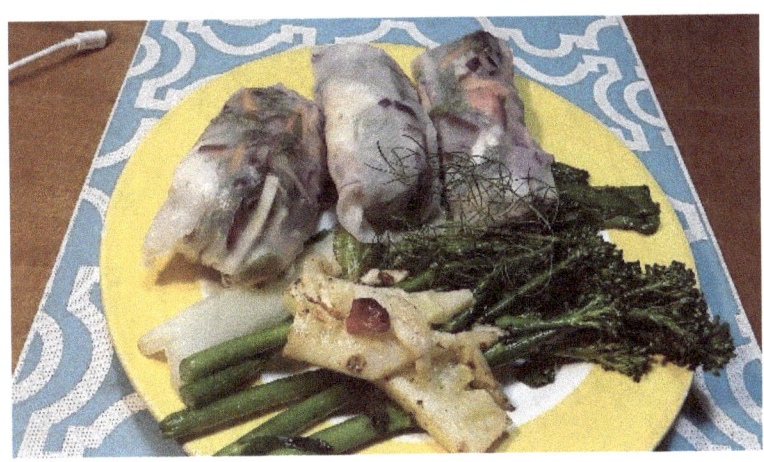

73. Hoki rolls, fried onion, asparagus

- 1 large Hoki fillet pan-fried in olive oil, cracked pepper, salt, sliced red onion, sambal oelek, asparagus **Use 3 rice paper rounds to make rolls**
- Pickled pink sushi ginger
- ¼ avocado, lime juice, coriander
- Greek yoghurt
- Cup of mixed coleslaw/Asian slaw, coriander
- Serve Hoki rolls with fried veges on the side.

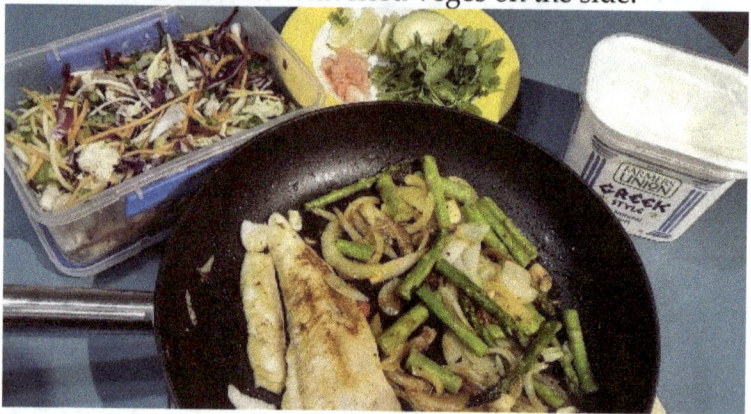

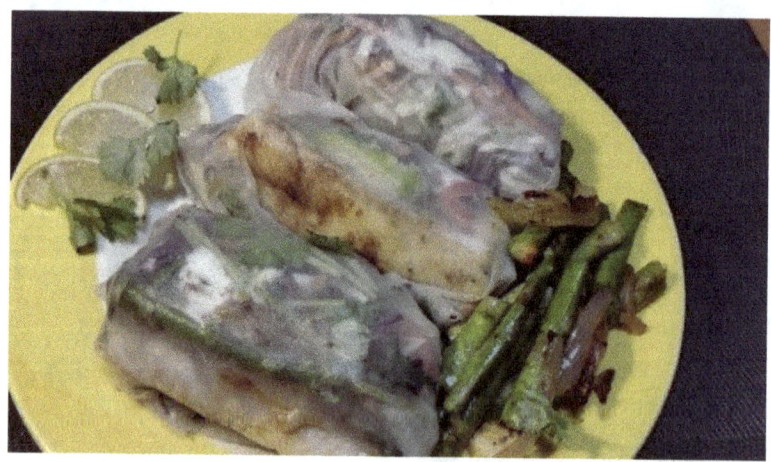

74. Pan-fried Hoki, balsamic salad

- To a hot pan, add olive oil, salt, pepper, thawed Hoki fillet, chopped sweet banana chili
- Add broccolini. Cook until stalks have softened.

In a serving bowl, add
- Cup of mixed lettuce leaves
- Cup of mixed American Coleslaw salad, with dressing
- Splash of balsamic vinegar
- Serve fish and cooked vegetables on top, with squeeze of lime juice. Season.

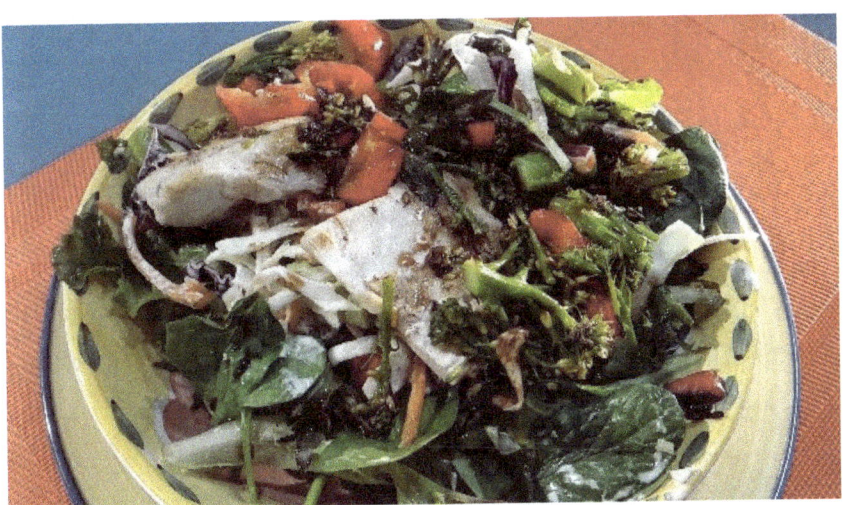

75. Steamed Hoki, prawns, Tom Yum

- To a hot pan, add drizzle olive oil, salt, cracked pepper, one heaped teaspoon Tom Yum Paste, one heaped teaspoon Tamarind Puree, fish sauce, ½ cup water
- Add mixed vegetables (broccoli, coleslaw, spinach, lettuce leaves). Stir.
- Add 1 frozen Hoki fillet and 100g frozen baby prawns
- Cover with lid. Cook until thick veges have softened.
- Serve in a bowl with lime juice.

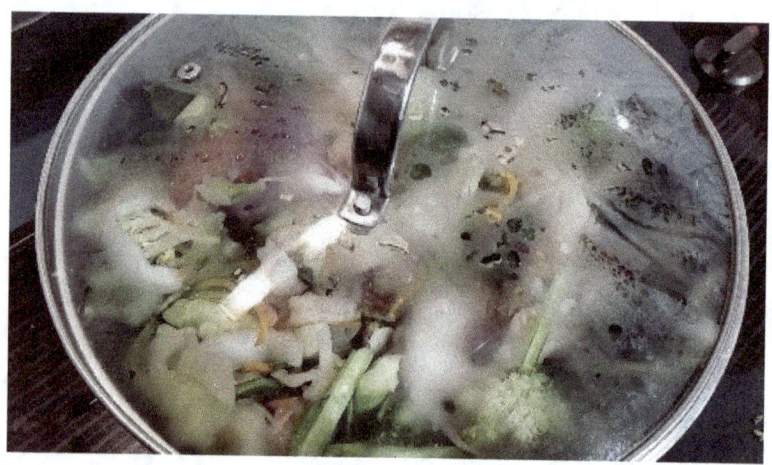

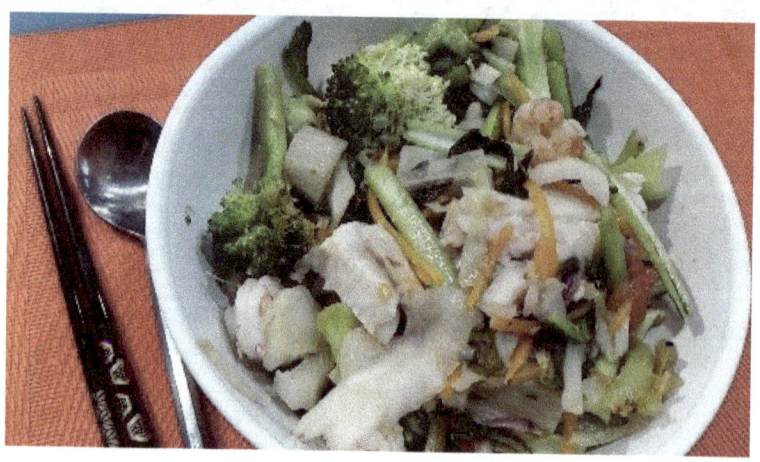

76. Steamed Hoki, curry, greens, avo

- To a hot pan, add chopped sweet banana chili, teaspoon hot red chili, tablespoon mild Yellow Curry Paste, ½ cup tinned tomatoes, ½ cup water, salt, cracked pepper
- Add broccoli, bok choy, handful of baby salad leaves.
- Add 2 thawed Hoki fillets
- Cover with lid. Cook until vegetables wilted.
  In a serving bowl, add
- ¼ avocado
- Cup of Southern Coleslaw, with spicy dressing
- Serve fish and cooked vegetables on top, with squeeze of lime juice. Season.

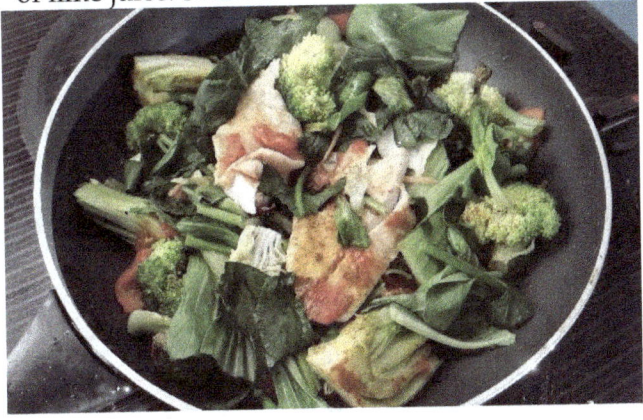

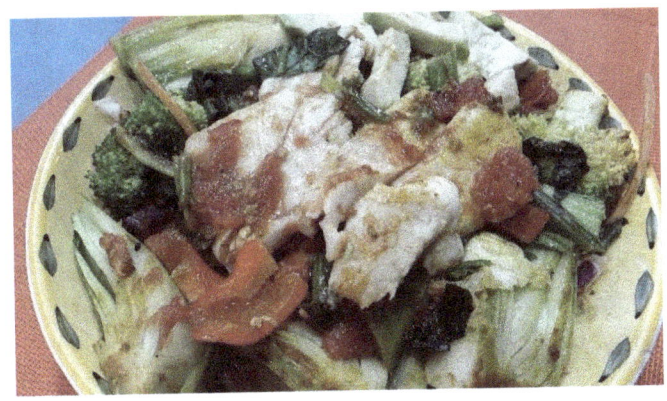

77. Steamed Hoki, Tom Yum, veg

- To a hot pan, add chopped sweet red banana chili, teaspoon hot red chili, large teaspoon Tom Yum Paste, ½ tin tomatoes, ½ cup water, salt, cracked pepper
- Add broccoli, broccolini, wombok, English spinach (or handful of baby salad leaves), cup mixed coleslaw veg
- Add 2 frozen Hoki fillets
- Cover with lid. Cook until thick veges have softened.
- Serve in a bowl with ¼ avocado, chopped Asian herbs, lime juice. Season.

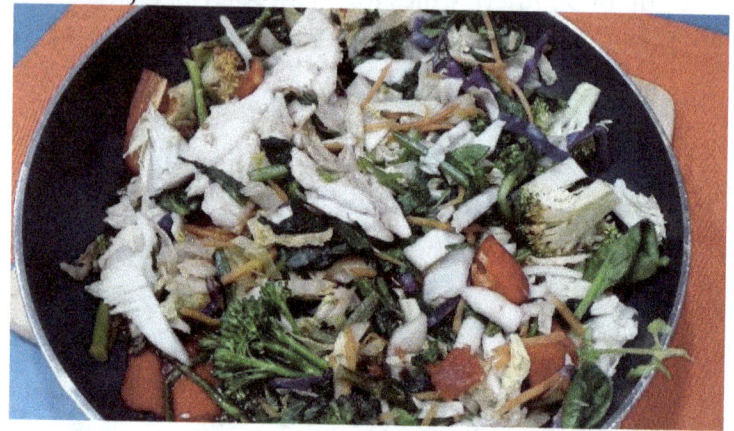

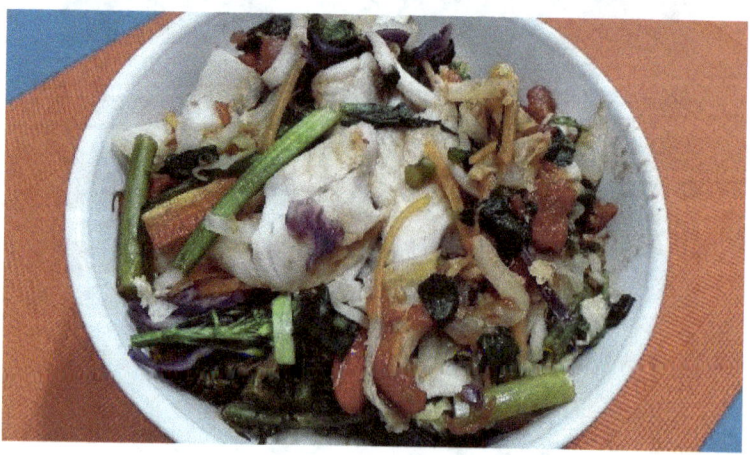

78. Steamed Hoki, Tamarind, Tom Yum

- To a hot pan, add drizzle olive oil, salt, cracked pepper, one heaped teaspoon Tom Yum Paste, one heaped teaspoon Tamarind Puree
- Add green vegetables (broccoli, bok choy, spinach)
- Stir.
- Add 2 frozen Hoki fish fillets
- Cover with lid. Cook until thick veges have softened.
- Serve in a bowl with lime juice. Season to taste with fish sauce and light soy sauce.

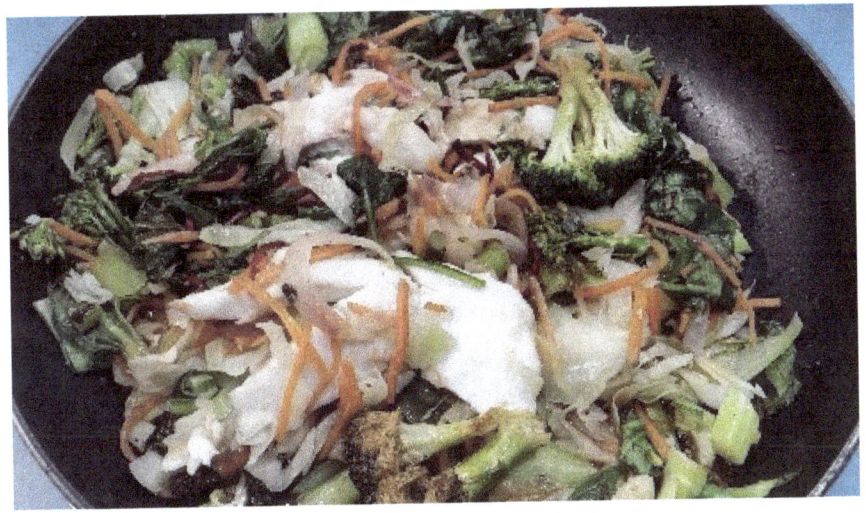

79. Steamed Hoki, peas, Tom Yum

- To a hot pan, add drizzle olive oil, salt, cracked pepper, one heaped teaspoon Tom Yum Paste, one heaped teaspoon Tamarind Puree
- Add broccoli, wombok, silverbeet, cup of coleslaw veg
- Add cup of frozen baby peas. Stir.
- Add 2 frozen Hoki fish fillets
- Cover with lid. Cook until thick veges have softened.
- Serve in a bowl with Greek yoghurt and your choice of Asian sauce, e.g. Ketjap Manis (sweet soy sauce).

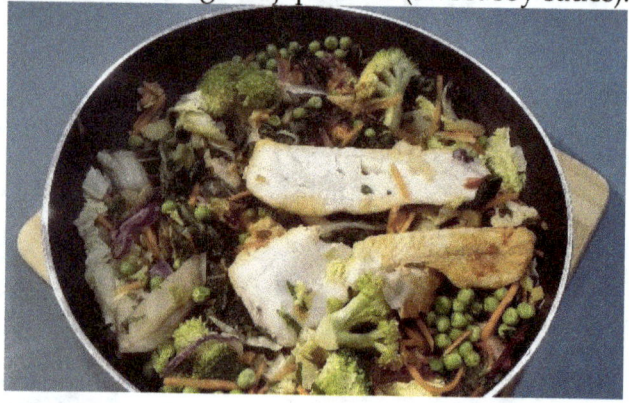

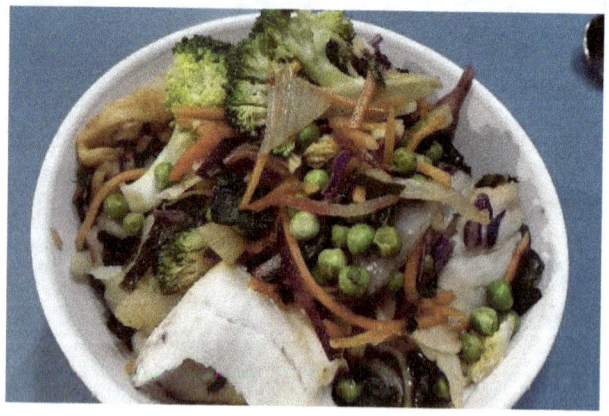

80. Hoki egg bacon pea scramble

- To a hot pan, add drizzle of olive oil, salt, cracked pepper, diced bacon, chopped chili, ½ cup frozen peas
- Add 2 thawed Hoki fish fillets, cut into chunks
- Add cup of mixed coleslaw veg.
- Beat 2 large free-range eggs, pour into pan. Give a little stir. Cover with lid.
- Cook for a couple of minutes until eggs have set.
- Serve in a bowl.
- Drizzle with Chang's Crispy Noodle Salad Dressing.

Sounds a bit wild and whacky, but the combination tastes good.

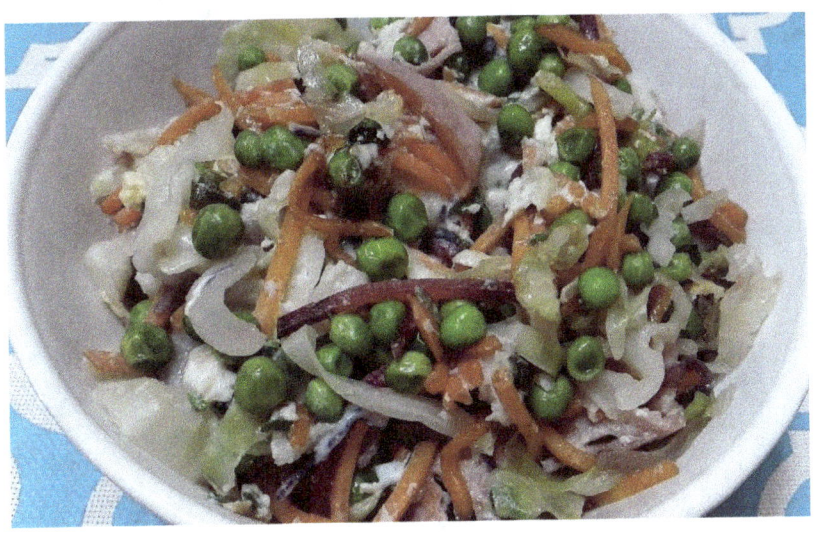

81. Braised Hoki, prawn, Tom Yum

- To a hot pan, add drizzle of olive oil, salt, cracked pepper, chopped sweet banana chili
- Add one heaped teaspoon Tom Yum Paste, ½ tin tomatoes, ½ cup water, splash of fish sauce. Stir.
- Add a frozen Hoki fillet, cut into chunks
- Add 100g frozen baby prawns
- Add vegetables (broccolini, cup of mixed coleslaw veg, cup of baby salad leaves). Stir.
- Cover with lid. Cook until broccolini stems soften.
- Serve in a bowl with mixed salad and lime juice.

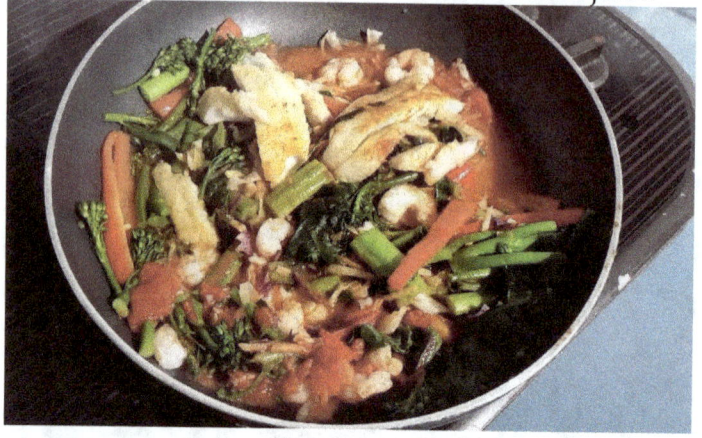

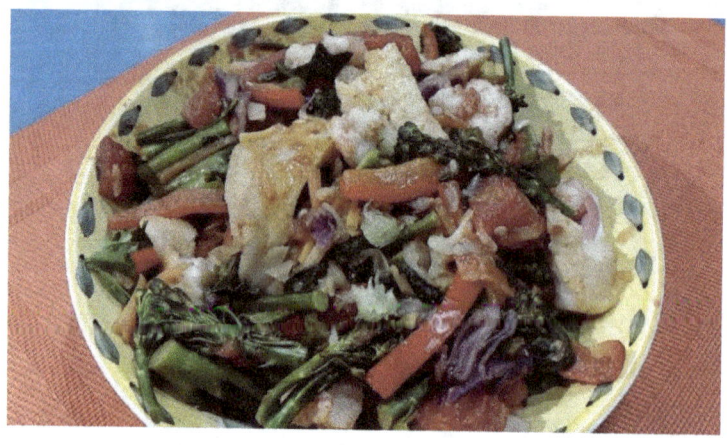

82. Braised Hoki Tom Yum, plum sauce

- To a hot pan, add drizzle of olive oil, salt, pepper
- Add sliced mushrooms, and fry until browned.
- Add splash of Plum Sauce
- Add a thawed Hoki fillet
- Add vegetables (cup of Rainbow Stir-fry veg, cup of kaleslaw, chopped broccoli)
- Add cup of water
- Cover with lid. Cook until broccoli stems soften.
- Balance seasoning with lemon juice, fish sauce, and sushi light soy sauce.

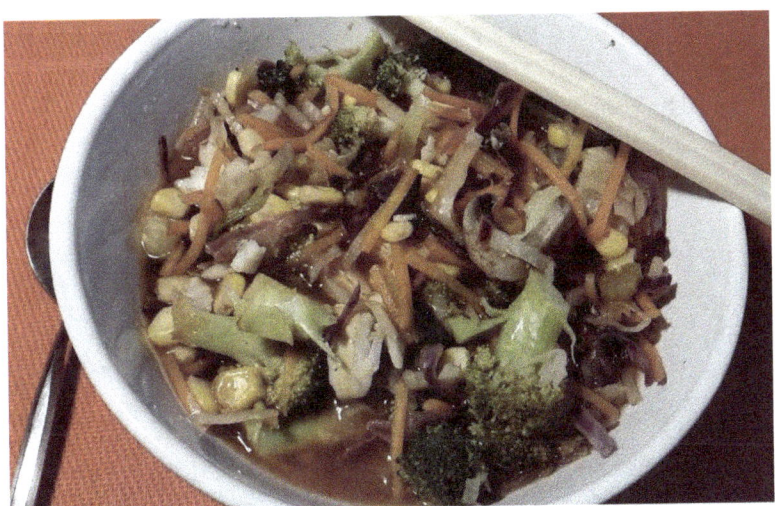

83. Hoki, onion, lemongrass noodle salad

- Add a serve of dried vermicelli noodles to a bowl and cover in boiling water. Leave for a few minutes. Stir to separate. Drain and set aside.

- To a hot pan, add drizzle of olive oil, salt, cracked pepper, garlic, chopped red chili, sliced red onion
  **Add frozen Hoki fillet and cook on both sides.
  In a serving bowl,**
- Cup of mixed coleslaw/kaleslaw/Asian salad kits
- Drained vermicelli noodles
- Fish and vegetables from pan
- Sliced fresh pineapple
- ¼ avocado
- Thai basil, fennel herb
- Vietnamese Lemongrass Salad Dressing
- Lime wedges. Season.

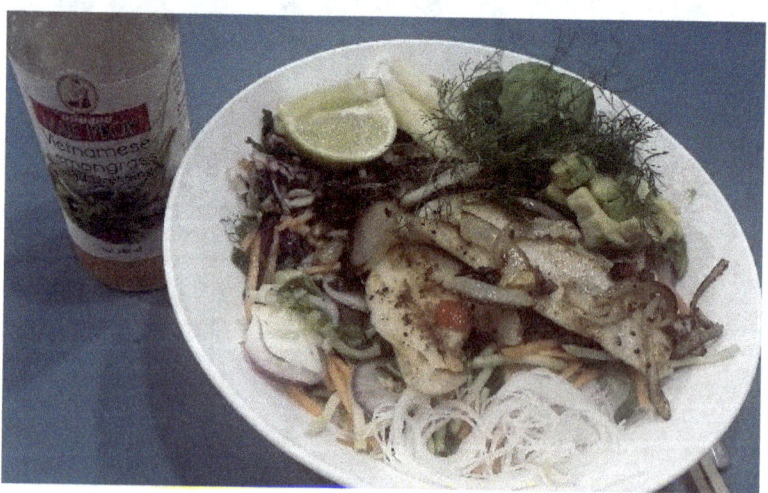

84. Hoki, garlic, fennel, avo, noodle bowl

- Reconstitute a serve of vermicelli noodles. Drain.
- To a hot pan, add olive oil, salt, pepper, teaspoon sambal oelek, 2 sliced garlic cloves, ½ sliced red onion
- Add ½ cup of thinly sliced fennel bulb
- Add chopped silverbeet, broccolini; cup of mixed coleslaw veg or stir-fry veg; cup of mixed salad leaves
- Add 2 frozen Hoki fillet.
- Cover with lid. Steam until broccolini stems soften.
- Add cooked vermicelli noodles to a serving bowl.
- Transfer everything from pan to a serving bowl.
- Finish with ½ avocado, pickled sushi ginger, squeeze lemon juice, drizzle Vietnamese Dipping Sauce
- Crunchy shallot flakes on top (from Asian salad kit)

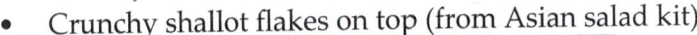

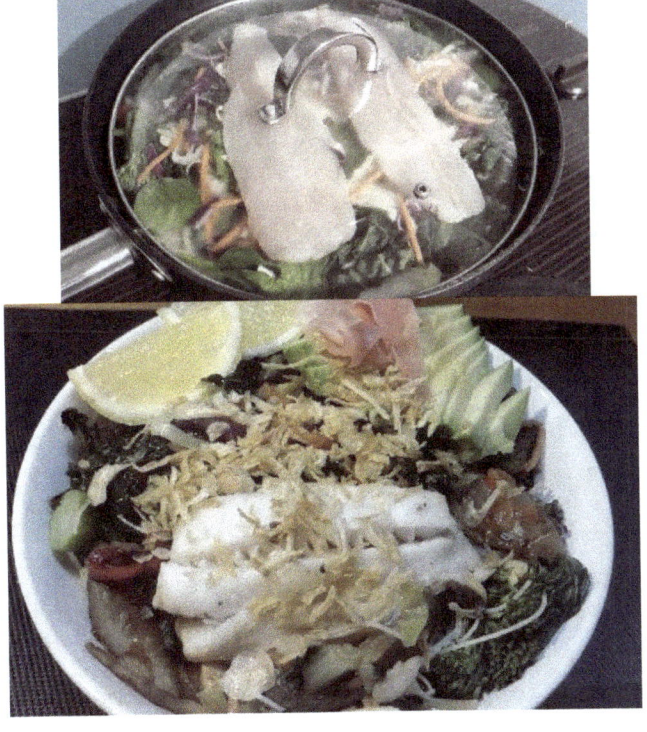

85. Hoki, Asian greens, Hoisin, noodle

- Reconstitute a serve of vermicelli noodles. Drain.
- To a hot pan, add olive oil, garlic, teaspoon sambal oelek
- Add 2 thawed Hoki fillets, season with salt
- Add leafy Asian greens (bok choy, gai lan, or choy sum)
- Add tablespoon Hoisin sauce, stir
- Add cooked noodles.
- Dissolve teaspoon of miso paste in ½ cup hot water. Add to pan. Cover with lid. Steam for a couple of minutes, until veges soften.
- Transfer to bowl. Finish with fresh lemon thyme.

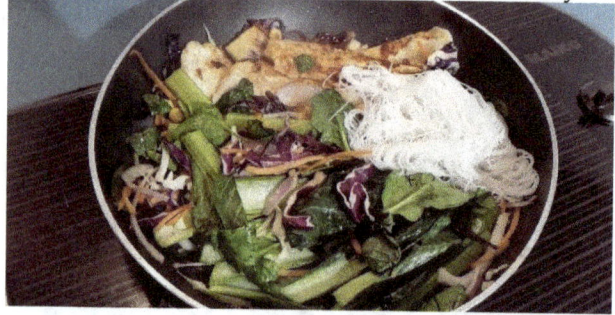

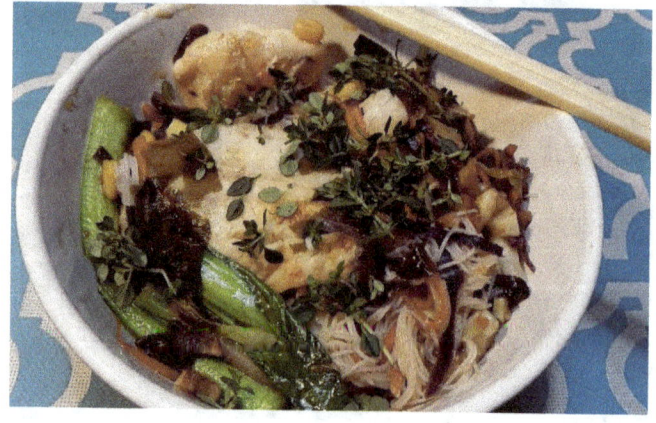

86. Hoki, mushroom, veg noodles

- Reconstitute a serve of vermicelli noodles. Drain.
- To a hot pan, add salt, cracked pepper, sliced mushrooms, and cook until browned.
- Add asparagus, chopped green chili, silverbeet
- Add a little olive oil, splash of fish sauce
- Add 2 thawed Hoki fillets. Pan-fry.
  In a serving bowl,
- Cup of kaleslaw (dry)
- Drained noodles
- Fish and vegetables from pan
- Pickled pink sushi ginger
- ¼ avocado
- Season with extra salt, pepper
- Drizzle with Thai Pineapple Salad Dressing

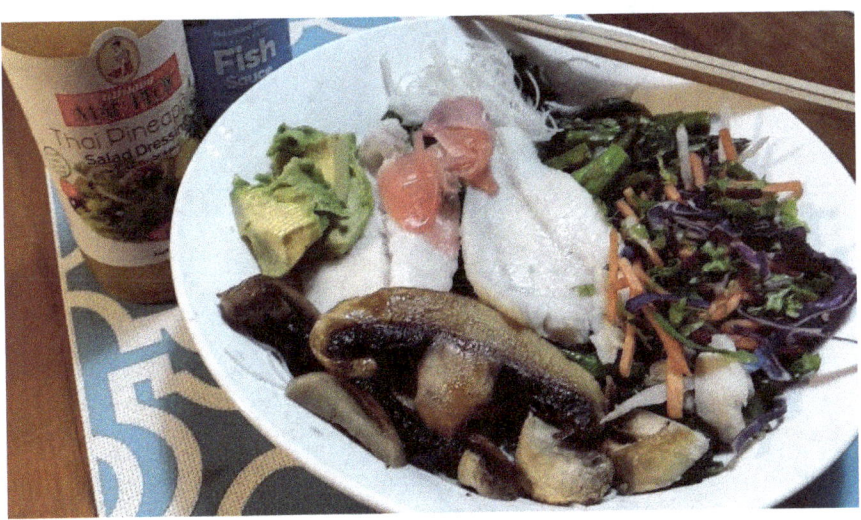

87. Hoki Tom Yum, chili, noodle soup

- Reconstitute a serve of vermicelli noodles. Drain.
- To a hot pan, add salt, cracked pepper, sliced mushrooms, and cook until browned.
- Add teaspoon Tom Yum paste, stir
- Add a little olive oil, teaspoon sambal oelek
- Add broccoli, bok choy, wombok, coleslaw veg
- Add thawed Hoki fillets and cover with baby leaf salad
- Add 4 ladles (about 2 cups) of boiling water
- Cover with lid. Cook until vegetables wilt down.
- Add drained noodles. Season.
- Transfer everything to a serving bowl, with lime wedges

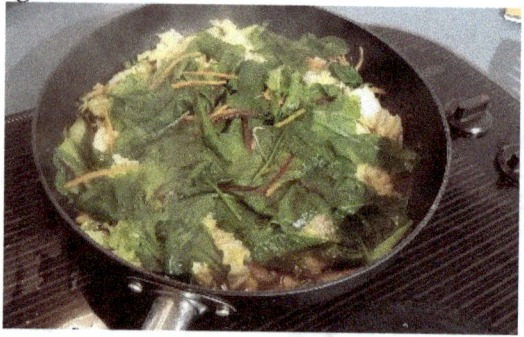

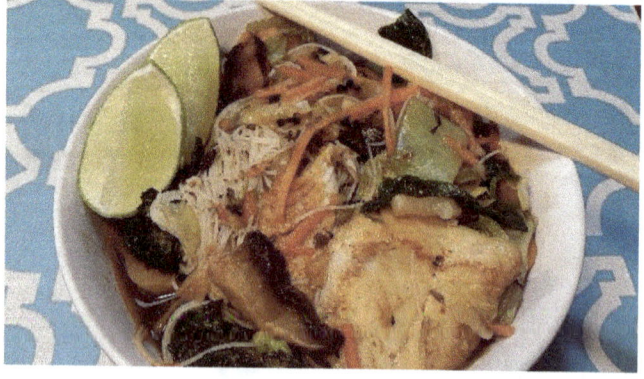

88. Hoki Tom Yum, Hoisin noodle soup

- Reconstitute a serve of vermicelli noodles. Drain.
- To a hot pan, add salt, cracked pepper, dessertspoon Tom Yum paste
- Add sliced mushrooms, broccoli, bok choy, wombok
- Add thawed Hoki fillets and cover with baby leaf salad
- Add splash of Hoisin sauce and fish sauce
- Add cup boiling water. Cover with lid. Cook until vegetables wilt down.
- Place drained noodles in a bowl. Top with cooked fish, veg, and juices from pan.
- Finish with coriander, Vietnamese mint, squeeze lime.

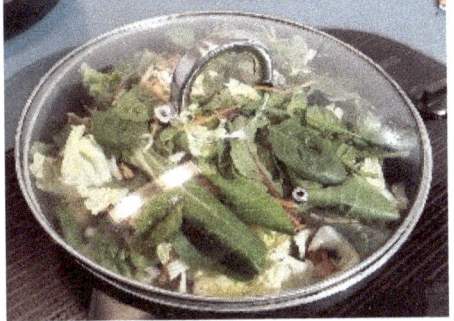

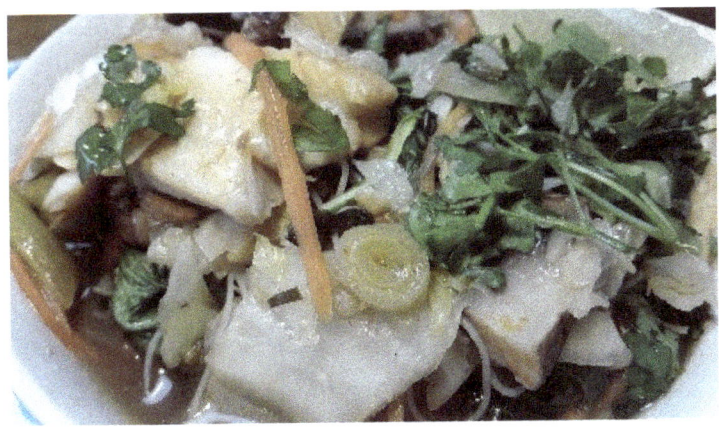

WHITING

There are many different whiting varieties, and they range in size. They are thin fillets with a very delicate flavour.

For these recipes, we used a particular brand of frozen whiting fillets which are sold in 1kg packs at Woolworths, and possibly elsewhere.

- **Just Caught** Whiting Fillets, skin on, 1kg packs

The packaging says they are Southern Blue Whiting, wild caught in New Zealand waters. They have skin on, but it is so thin that you hardly notice it.

89. Whiting rolls, passata curry

- In hot pan, stir-fry olive oil, sambal oelek, tomato passata, teaspoon curry powder or paste, ½ cup coleslaw veg, salt, pepper.
- Add thawed whiting fillet. Cook both sides.
- Allow fish to cool slightly, or heat will turn rice papers to mush. Serve in 3 rice paper rolls, with Greek yoghurt, and cup of mixed coleslaw/kaleslaw

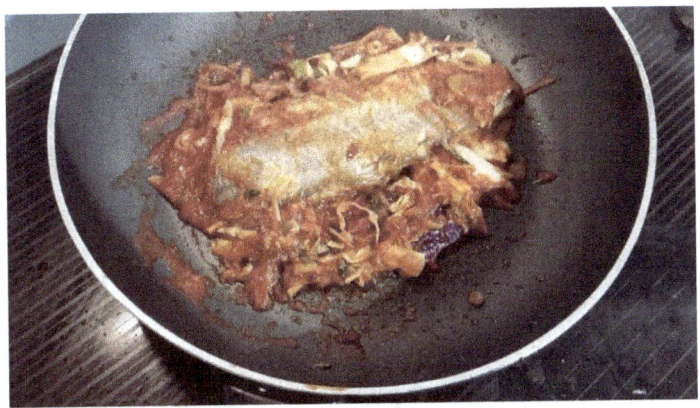

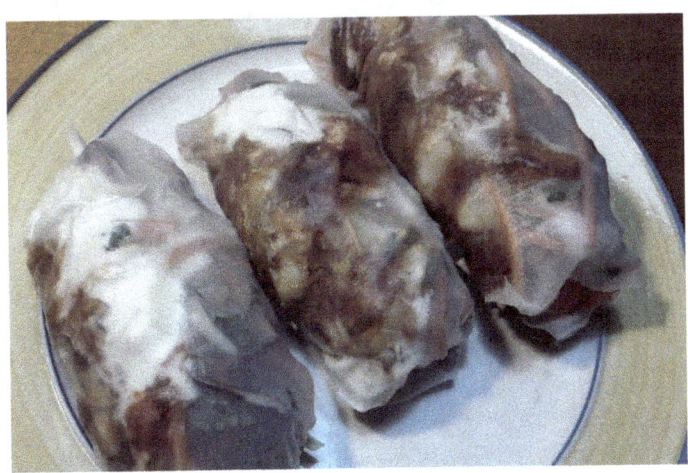

90. Whiting rolls, chili, green beans

- In hot pan, stir-fry olive oil, splash of hot sauce, fresh green beans, salt, pepper
- Add thawed whiting fillet. Cook both sides.
- Allow to cool slightly, or heat will turn rice papers to mush.

Serve in 3 rice paper rolls, with beans on the side

- ¼ avocado, fresh chili, coriander
- Cup crunchy coleslaw with spicy Asian salad dressing
- ½ sheet nori seaweed, snipped

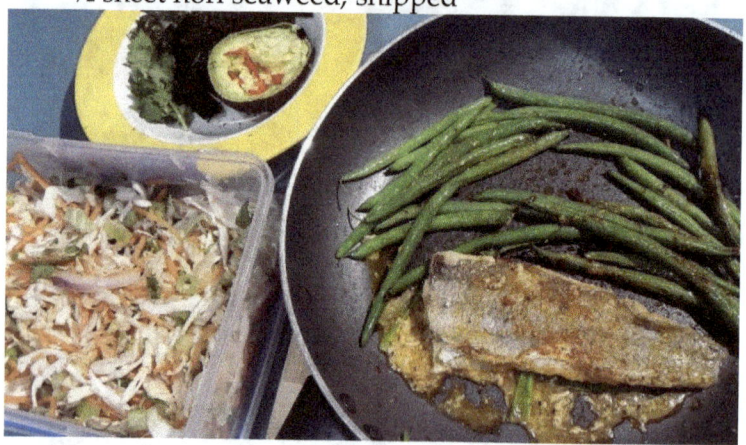

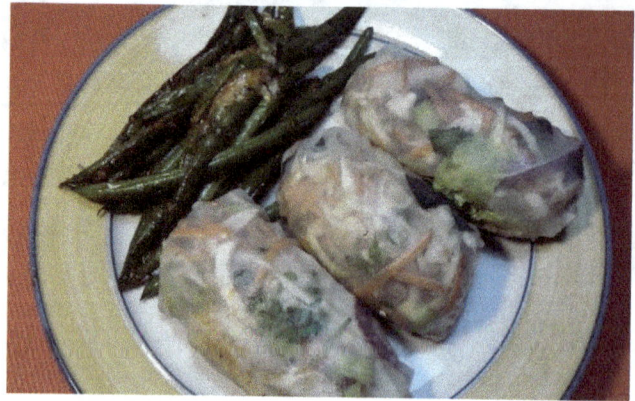

91. Pan-fried whiting, chili, soy, sesame bowl

- To a hot pan, add olive oil, sesame oil, sambal oelek, cracked pepper, splash of light soy sauce.
- Add frozen whiting fillet. Pan-fry both sides.
  In a serving bowl,
- Cup of mixed coleslaw/mesculin salad (dry)
- ¼ avocado, chopped shallot
- Pickled pink sushi ginger, sliced jalapenos
- Vietnamese Dipping Sauce
- Add cooked fish. Salt. Dollop of Greek yoghurt

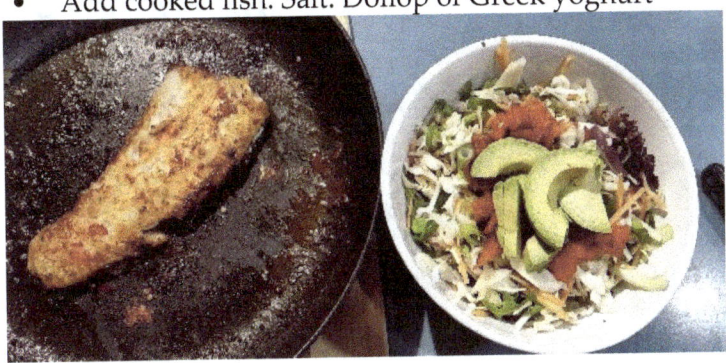

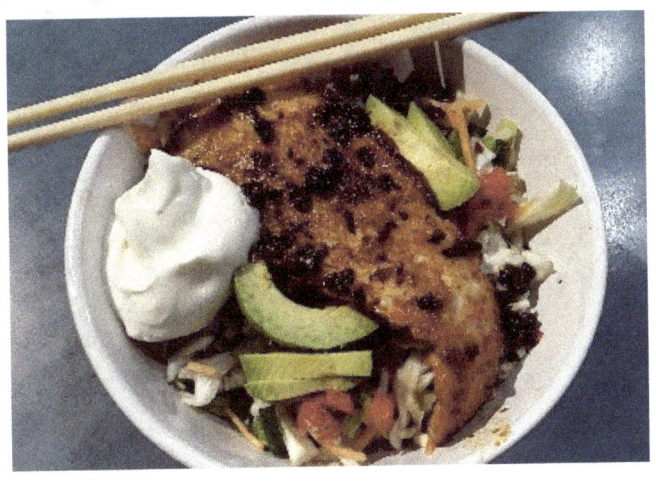

92. Whiting, wombok, Tom Yum soup

- Pan-fry frozen whiting fillet in hot pan, with olive oil, sliced red onion, sliced tomato, teaspoon Tom Yum Paste, salt
- Add bok choy, wombok, cup of coleslaw veg, cup of mixed baby leaves, juice of one lemon, cup of hot water
- Add herbs (parsley, fennel, Viet mint)
- Stir, cover with lid, and cook for a minute.
- Transfer everything to a serving bowl.

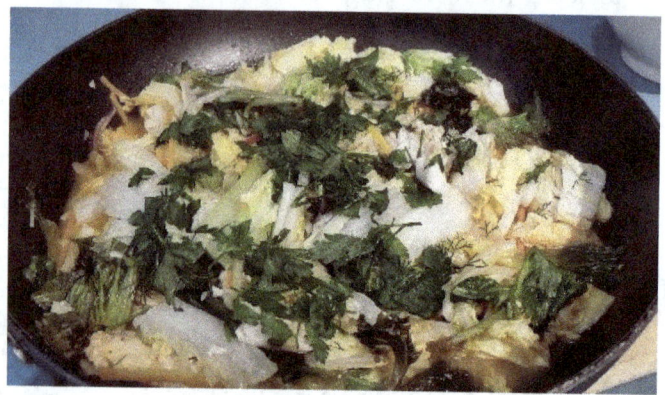

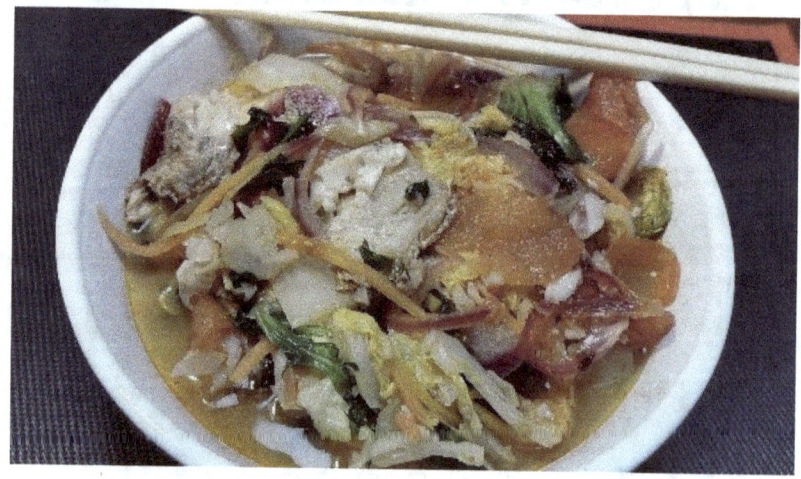

93. Whiting, tomato, Tom Yum noodles

- Reconstitute a serve of vermicelli noodles. Drain.
- Pan-fry frozen whiting fillet in hot pan, with olive oil, chopped shallots, teaspoon Tom Yum Paste, large teaspoon Tamarind Puree, salt, pepper
- Add sliced mushrooms, broccoli, cup of coleslaw veg
- Mix ½ cup tomato passata, ½ tin tomato pieces, ½ cup water. Pour over fish.
- Add drained noodles. Cover with lid. Steam for a couple of minutes. Transfer everything to a serving bowl.

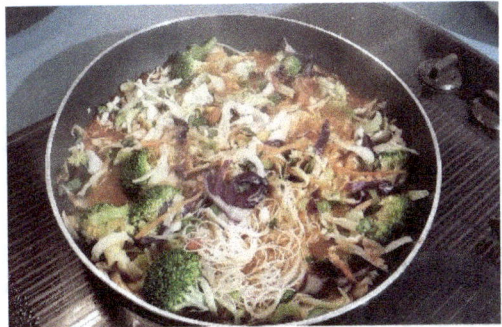

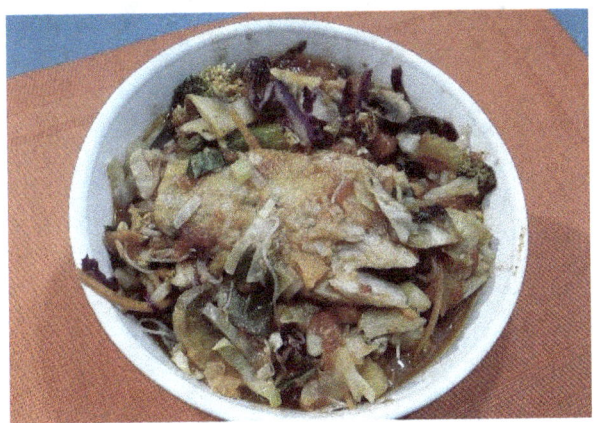

94. Whiting, tomato, peas, noodle soup

- Reconstitute a serve of vermicelli noodles. Drain.
- Pan-fry frozen whiting fillet in hot pan, with olive oil, chopped shallots, teaspoon Tom Yum Paste, large teaspoon Tamarind Puree, salt, cracked pepper
- Add sliced mushrooms, ½ cup frozen peas, cup of coleslaw veg
- Mix ½ cup tomato passata, ½ tin tomato pieces, ½ cup water. Pour over fish.
- Add drained noodles. Cover with lid. Steam for a couple of minutes. Add juice of one lime.
- Transfer everything to serving bowl.

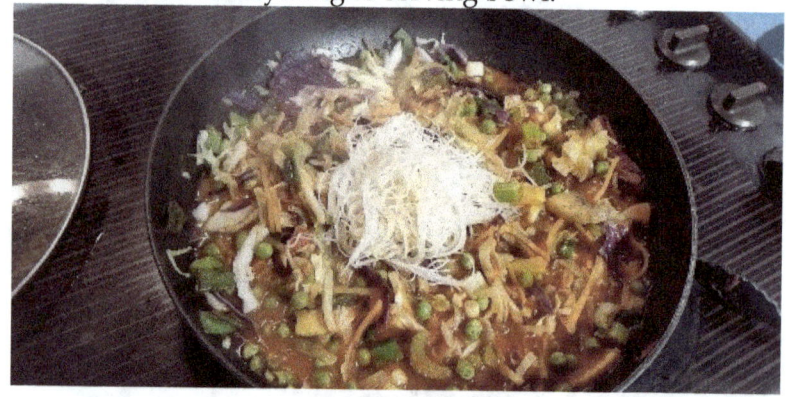

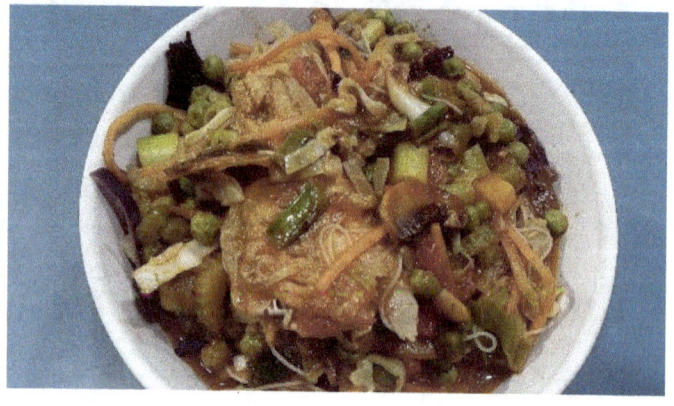

BARRAMUNDI

Barramundi and other thick fish should be cooked until the middle is opaque white, ready to give way, but not falling apart.

Wild-caught fresh barramundi has the best flavour and texture, but is rarely available these days. It is best steamed or lightly pan-fried.

The 'fresh' barramundi sold in supermarkets and fish shops is generally 'farmed' – often in Australia, but the cheapest fillets are often imported from farms in Asia. This is what you will find in most restaurants.

Packs of individually wrapped frozen portions can be stored in the freezer for convenience, and they are economical too. Especially suited to soups and stews.

95. Barra rolls, avo, sambal oelek

- Thawed barra fillet pan-fried in olive oil, cracked pepper, salt
- Allow to cool a little before making rice paper rolls. **Use 3 rice paper rounds to make rolls**
- Add cooked barra fillet
- Teaspoon Sambal oelek
- ¼ avocado
- Greek yoghurt
- Cup of coleslaw, with dressing
- Vietnamese mint

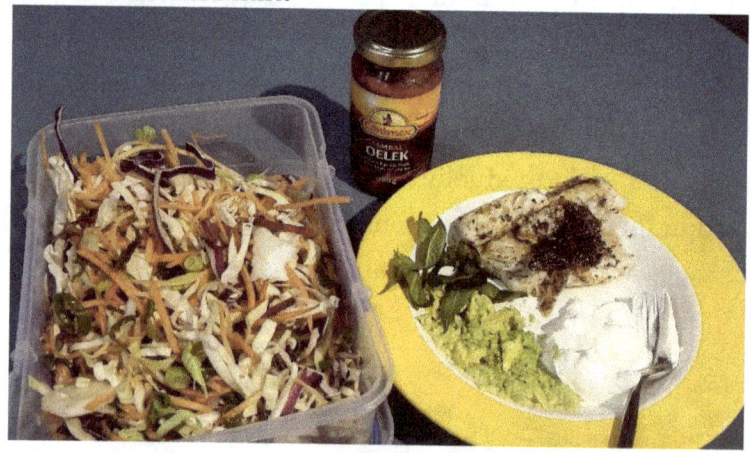

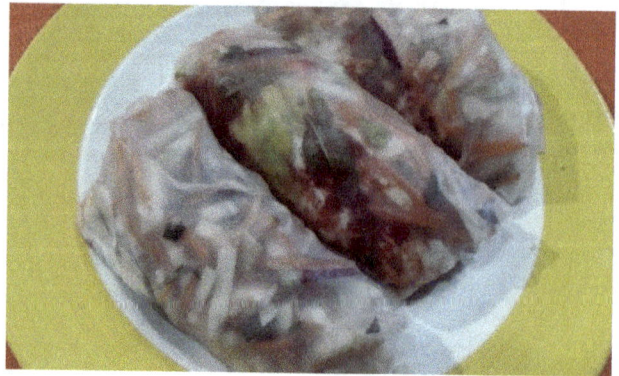

96. Barra rolls, Asian greens, avo

- Thawed barra fillet pan-fried in olive oil, cracked pepper, salt
- Pan-fry vegetables in same pan (broccolini, bok choy)
- Allow to cool a little before attempting rice paper rolls. **Use 3 rice paper rounds to make rolls**
- Add cooked barra fillet
- Chopped chili
- ¼ avocado
- Greek yoghurt
- Cup of mixed coleslaw (dry)
- Serve cooked vegetables on the side.

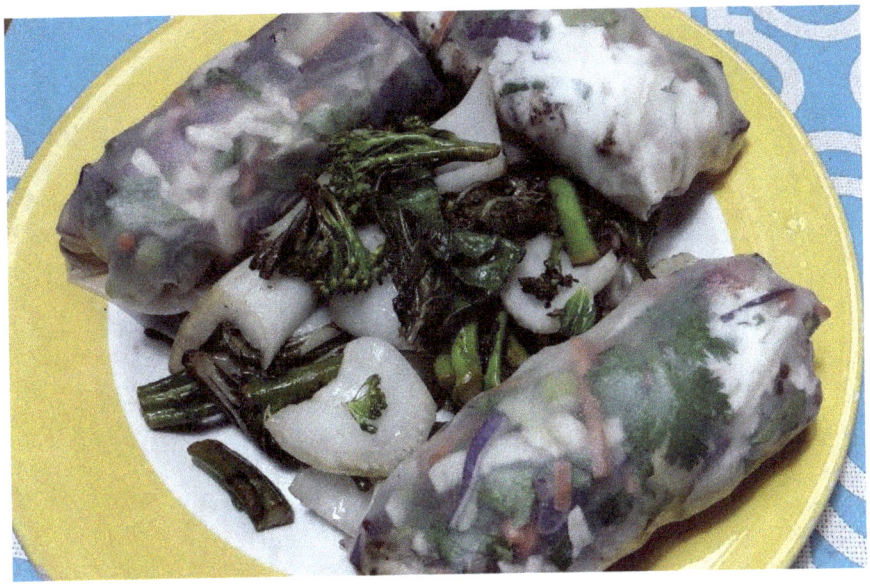

97. Avo rolls, spicy fried barra, greens

- Pan-fry chopped green chili in hot pan with olive oil
- Add chopped vegetables (broccolini, silverbeet)
- Add thawed barra fillet, pan-fry both sides until just cooked. Season with salt and cracked pepper.
  Make 2 rice paper rolls with salad
- Cos lettuce
- ¼ avocado
- Greek yoghurt
- Cup of mixed coleslaw (dry), alfalfa sprouts
- Serve cooked fish and vegetables on the side.

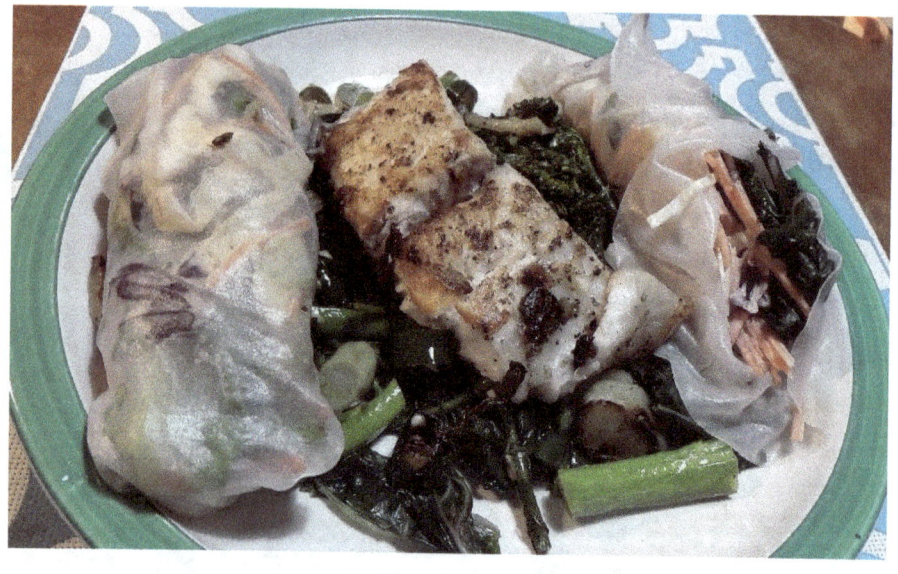

98. Pan-fried barra, garlic, capsicum, avo

- To a hot pan, add olive oil, garlic, strips of oven-roasted red capsicum, chopped bok choy
- Add fresh barramundi fillet (skinless). Season salt, cracked pepper. Pan-fry both sides.
  In a serving bowl,
- Cup of crunchy coleslaw salad (dry)
- Add cooked barra and vegetables
- ¼ avocado, lime juice, chopped red chili
- Greek yoghurt
- Pickled pink sushi ginger

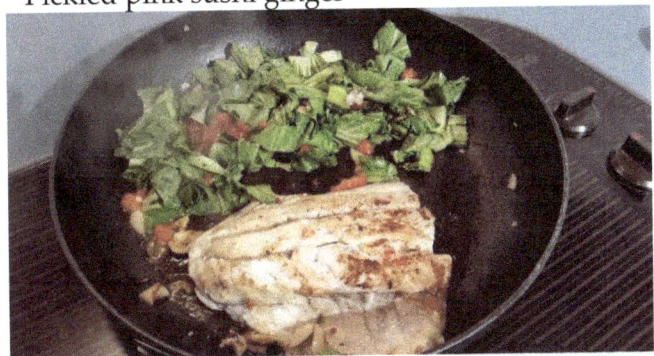

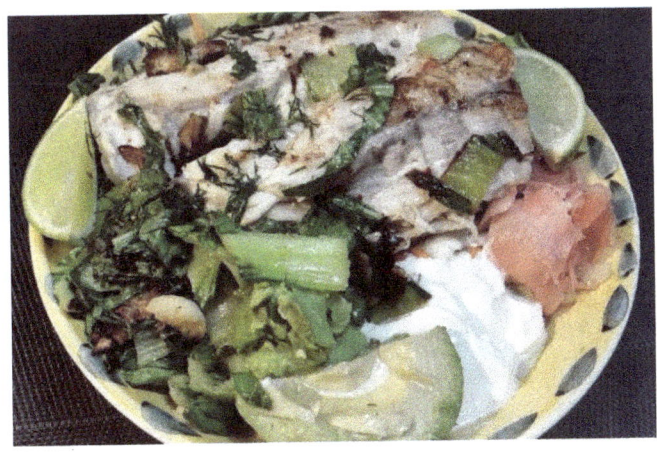

99. Pan-fried barra, capers, beetroot bowl

- To a hot pan, add olive oil, sesame oil, teaspoon sambal oelek, capers, chopped leafy Asian greens (gai lan or choy sum)
- Add fresh barramundi fillet (skinless). Season salt, cracked pepper. Pan-fry both sides until just cooked.
  In a serving bowl,
- Cup of crunchy coleslaw salad (with dressing)
- Add cooked barra, vegetables, and fried capers on top
- Pickled pink sushi ginger
- Sliced beetroot, dollop of Greek yoghurt

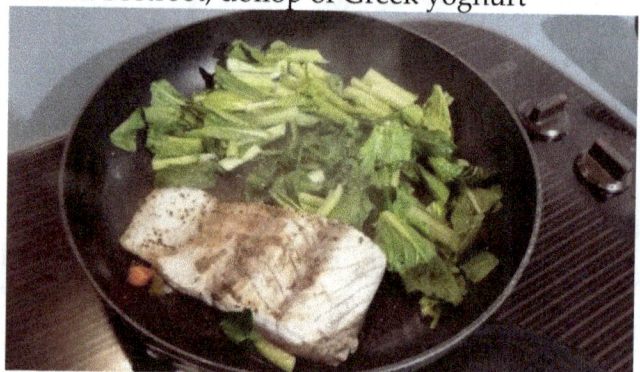

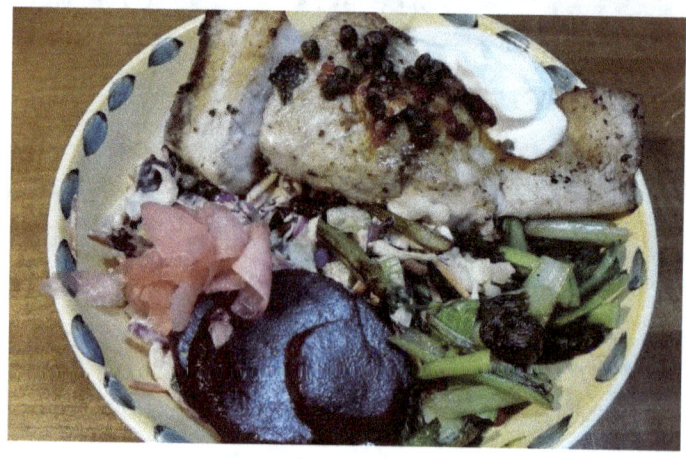

100. Braised wild barramundi, veg bowl

- To a hot pan, add drizzle of olive oil, sliced red onion, teaspoon grated fresh ginger, sweet red banana chili
- Add a fillet of FRESH barramundi (skinless). Pan-fry both sides. Salt, pepper.
- Add vegetables (shredded wombok, chopped silverbeet, cup of coleslaw veg, Thai basil, Viet mint)
- Add ½ cup of hot water. Season veges. Cover with lid. Steam until fish is cooked. Squeeze of lemon juice.

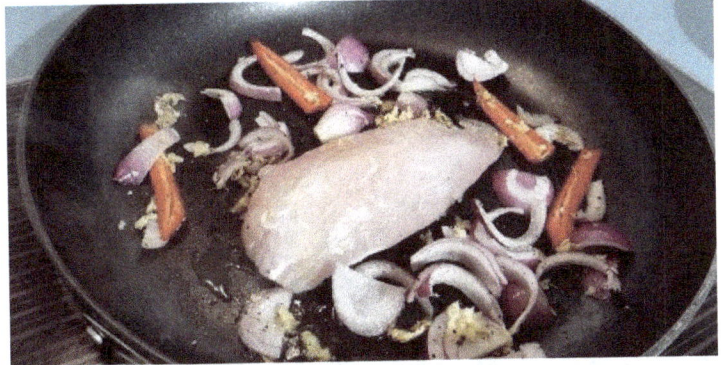

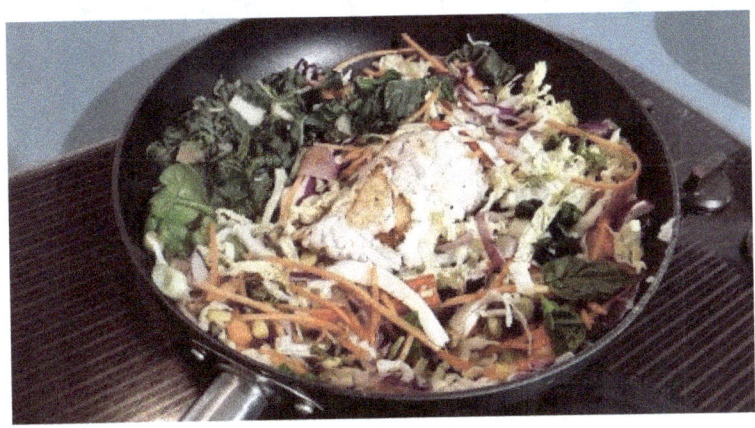

101. Braised barra, passata, veg bowl

- To a hot pan, add olive oil, teaspoon Tom Yum Paste, habanero mild chili, salt, cracked pepper
- Add sliced mushrooms. Fry until browned.
- Add partially-thawed barra fillet (skinless). Pan-fry.
- Add vegetables (spinach, coleslaw, shredded wombok)
- Mix ½ cup tomato passata, ½ tin tomato pieces, ½ cup water. Pour over fish.
- Cover with lid. Steam for a couple of minutes until fish cooked. Serve with juice of one lime.

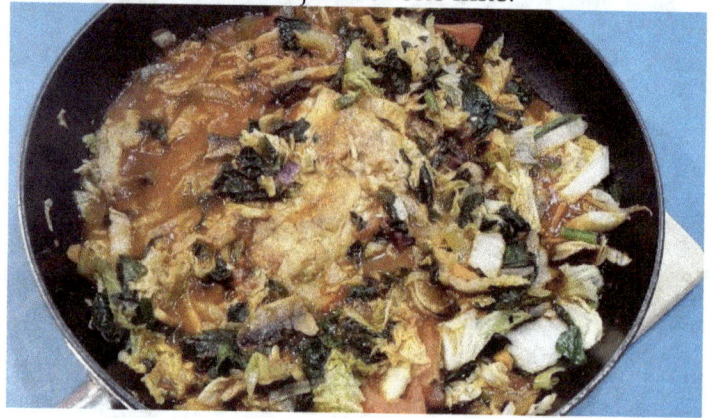

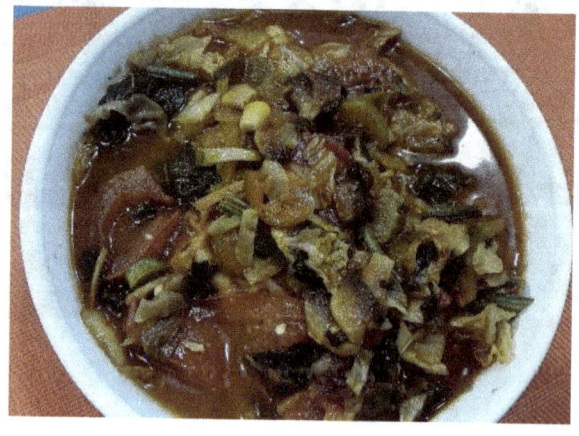

102. Braised barra, bok choy, soup bowl

- **NB: Double the usual quantity – enough for dinner and lunch next day.**
- To a hot pan, add olive oil, teaspoon sambal oelek chili paste, mild red banana chili, salt, cracked pepper
- Add sliced mushrooms. Fry until browned.
- Add 2 partially-thawed barra fillet (skinless). Pan-fry.
- Add vegetables (bok choy, spinach, coleslaw, wombok)
- Mix 1 cup tomato passata, tin of tomato pieces, cup of water. Pour over fish.
- Cover with lid. Steam for a couple of minutes until fish cooked. Adjust seasonings with lime juice, light soy sauce, and/or fish sauce, as desired. Add Asian herbs.

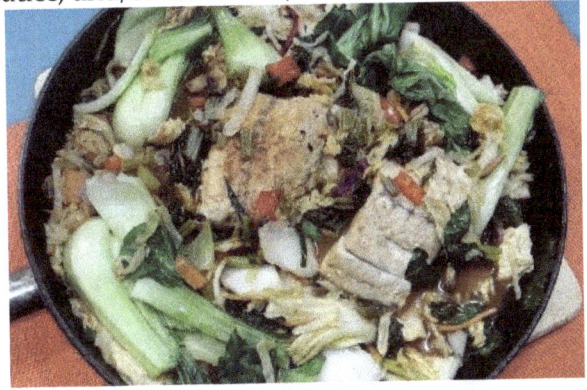

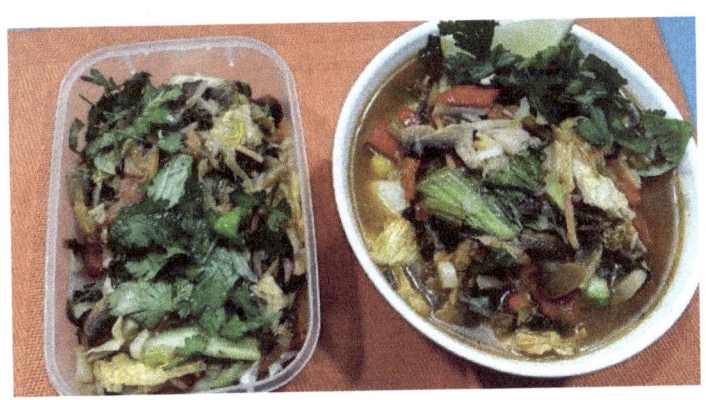

103. Barramundi PHO soup

- To a hot pan, add olive oil, salt, cracked pepper, green chili, a little fresh rosemary
- Add vegetables (broccoli, baby bok choy, cup of mixed stir-fry veg)
- Add partially-thawed barra fillet (skinless), cut into goujons (finger-sized strips).
- Add teaspoon Tom Yum paste
- Add teaspoon **Ayam** Vietnamese PHO soup paste
- Add cup of hot water
- Cover with lid. Simmer for 2-3 minutes.
- Transfer to a bowl. Adjust seasonings with lime juice, light soy sauce, and/or fish sauce, as desired.

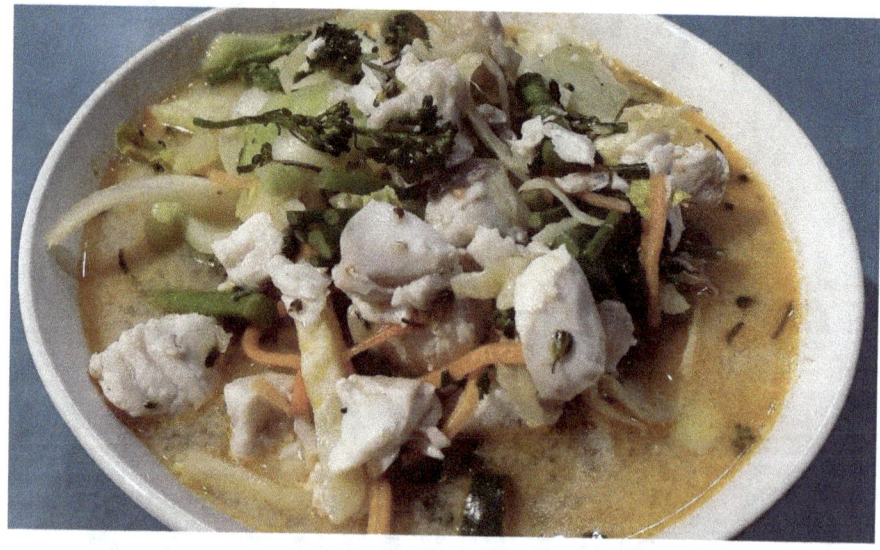

104. Crispy skin barra, dill, rolls

- 1 x partially-thawed barra fish fillet, skin on
- Pan-fry barra in hot pan, with oil, salt, pepper, and broccolini
- Follow instructions at the front of this book, for HOW TO COOK CRISPY SKIN FISH. Allow to cool a little before making these rice paper rolls.
- **Use 3 rice paper rounds to make rolls**
- Pickled pink sushi ginger
- Cup of mixed coleslaw, with dressing
- Dill.
- Add cooked barra fillet (warm)
- Serve with crispy skin on the side.

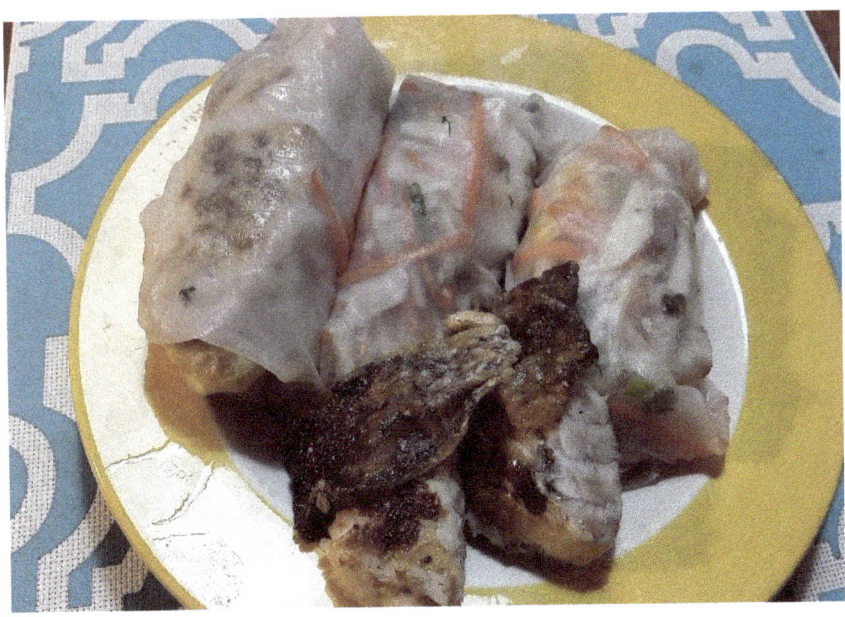

105. Crispy skin barra, ginger, rolls

- 1 x partially-thawed barra fish fillet, skin on
- Follow instructions at the front of this book, for HOW TO COOK CRISPY SKIN FISH.
- Pan-fry barra accordingly, in hot pan, with oil, salt, pepper, and grated fresh ginger
- Allow to cool a little before making these rice paper rolls.
  Use 3 rice paper rounds to make rolls
- Asian salad mix (dry)
- Vietnamese Dipping sauce for spring rolls
- Add cooked barra fillet (warm)
- Tartare Sauce
- Serve barra rolls with crispy skin on the side.

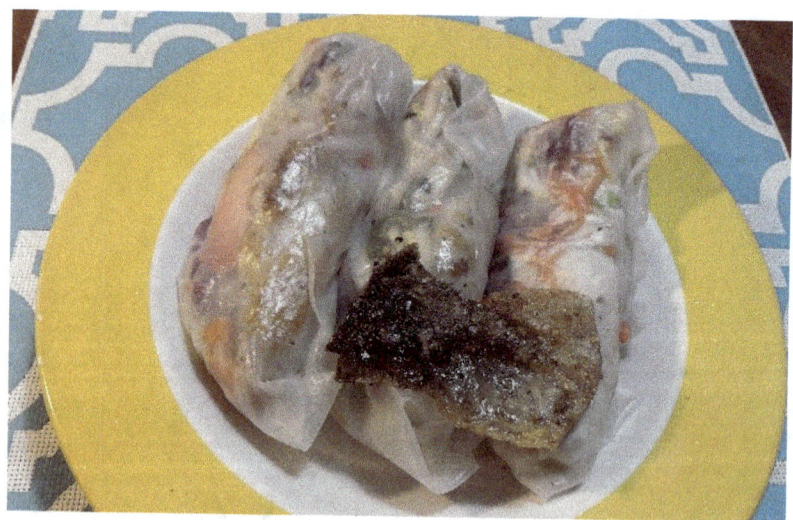

106. Crispy skin barra, salad bowl

- 1 x partially-thawed barra fish fillet, skin on
- Pan-fry barra in hot pan, with oil, salt, pepper, and broccolini
- Follow instructions at the front of this book, for HOW TO COOK CRISPY SKIN FISH.
- In a serving bowl, add
- Cup of mixed coleslaw
- Cup baby salad leaves
- Alfalfa sprouts
- ¼ avocado
- Greek yoghurt
- Chopped shallot, dill
- Top with cooked fish, crispy skin, and broccolini

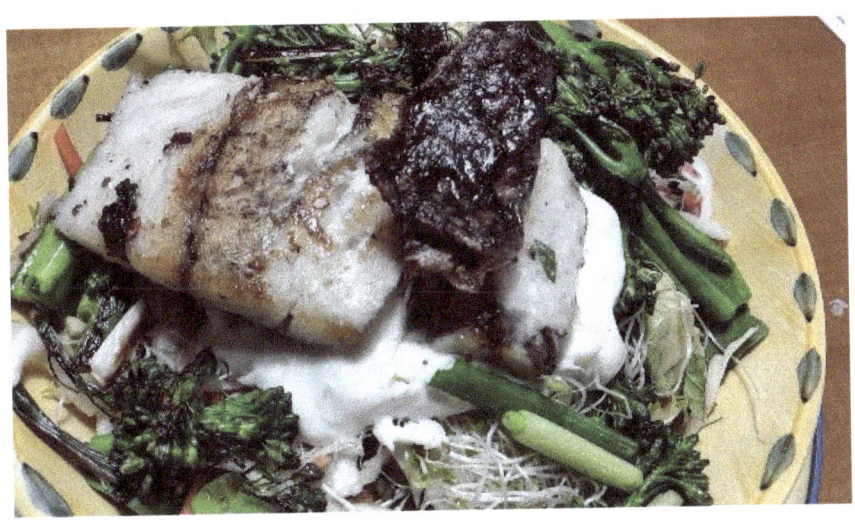

107.   Pan-fried barra, tomato, noodle bowl

- Reconstitute a serve of vermicelli noodles. Drain and chill.
- Pan-fry partially-thawed barra fillet (skinless) in hot pan, with olive oil, salt, cracked pepper
  In a serving bowl,
- Cup of crunchy coleslaw salad (with dressing)
- Transfer rice noodles to bowl
- Transfer cooked barramundi to bowl
- Sliced fresh tomato
- Pickled pink sushi ginger
- Sliced jalapenos
- Drizzle Vietnamese Dipping Sauce

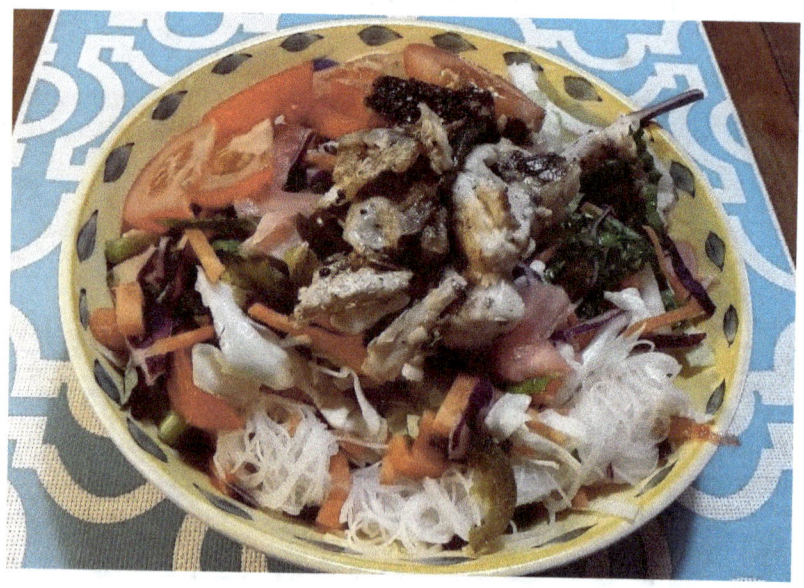

RED EMPEROR

Red Emperor is one of Australia's most popular reef fish. It has firm white flesh, large flake, and delicate flavour. Ideal accompaniment to Asian flavours.

The moist flesh is well suited to a variety of cooking methods, such as steaming, poaching, grilling or pan frying.

108. Crispy skin Red Emperor rolls

- 1 x fresh RED EMPEROR fish fillet, skin on
- Follow instructions at the front of this book, for HOW TO COOK CRISPY SKIN FISH. Allow to cool a little before making these rice paper rolls.
- 3 rice paper rounds
- Jalapenos, picked chili
- Cup of mixed coleslaw/kaleslaw, with dressing
- Mixed lettuce leaves. Thai basil.
- Serve with crispy skin on the side.

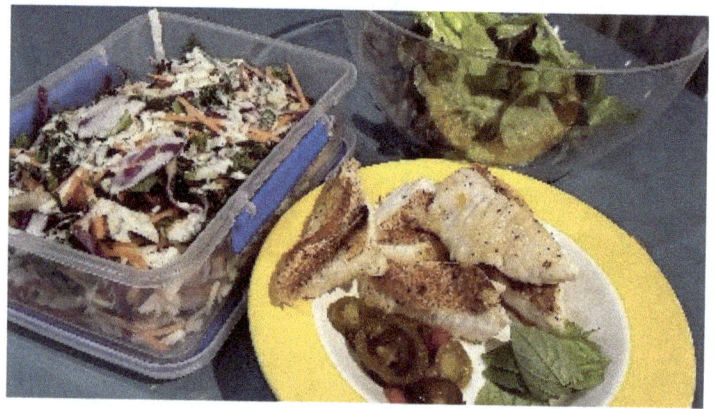

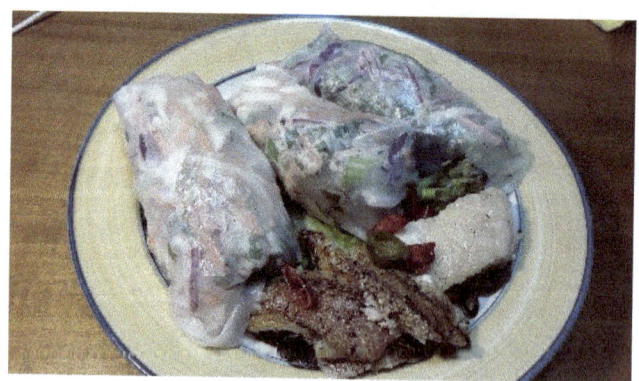

NORWEGIAN TROUT

Norwegian Trout is similar to salmon in flavour, but usually cheaper. Like salmon, it has a dense, firm protein structure which holds up well to pan-frying, grilling, or baking.

109. Crispy skin trout, nori, rolls

- To a hot pan, add olive oil, sesame oil, red chili
- Add fillet of fresh Norwegian Trout (skin-side down).
- Follow instructions at front of this book, for HOW TO COOK CRISPY SKIN FISH. Season with salt, pepper.
- Allow fish to cool a little before making the rice paper rolls, or the papers will go soft and mushy.
  Use 3 rice paper rounds to make rolls:
- Mixed coleslaw/kaleslaw (dry)
- Sliced trout (warm)
- Pickled pink sushi ginger
- ½ sheet nori seaweed
- Greek yoghurt
- Vietnamese mint, fennel, parsley
- Serve with lemon wedges and crispy skin on the side.

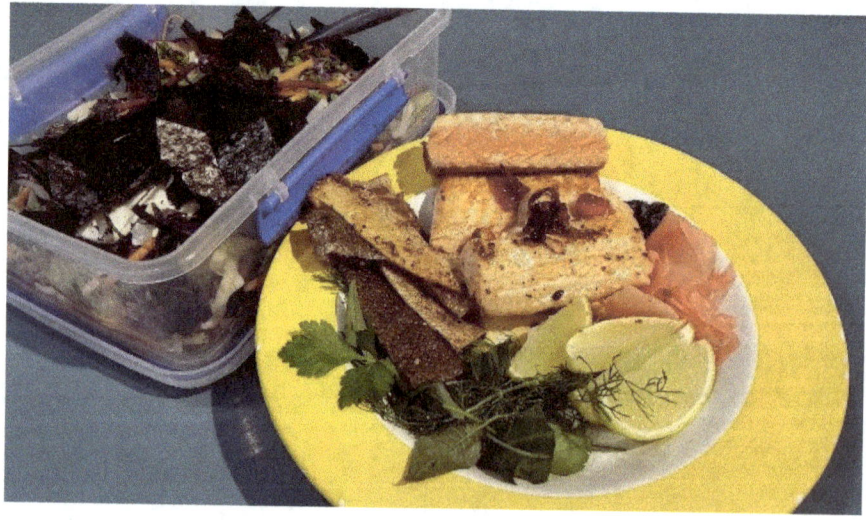

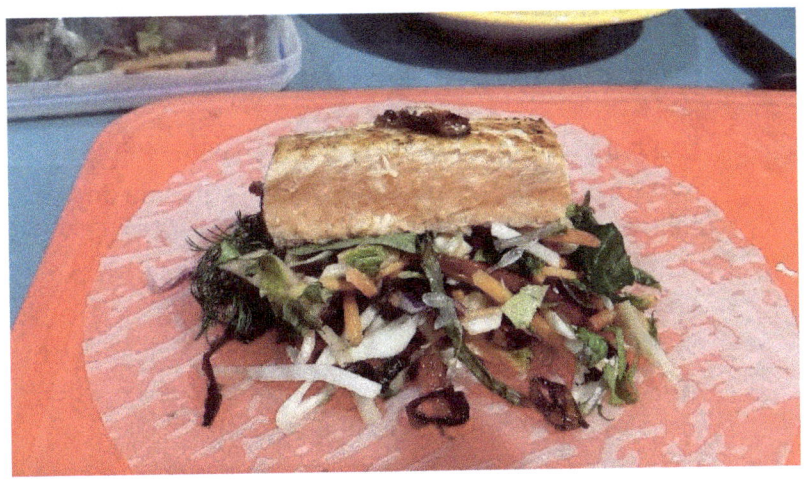

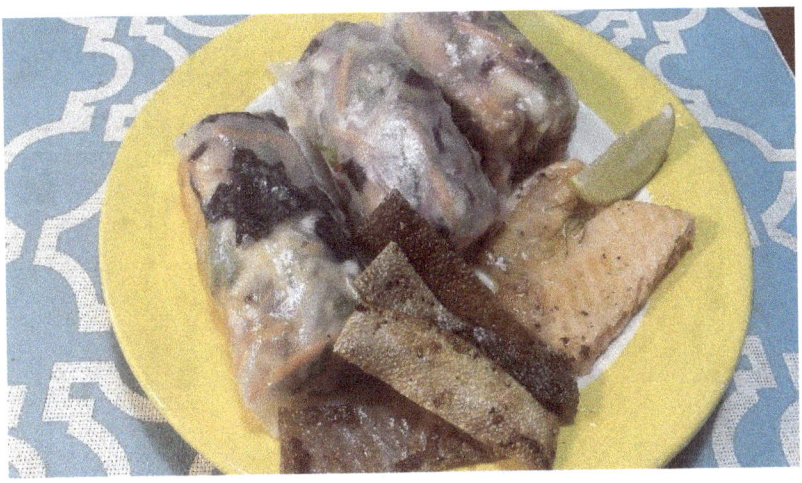

110. Crispy skin trout, garlic, fried veg, rolls

- To a hot pan, add olive oil, garlic, red chili
- Add fillet of fresh Norwegian Trout (skin-side down).
- Follow instructions at front of this book, for HOW TO COOK CRISPY SKIN FISH. Season with salt, pepper.
- Add vegetables (silverbeet, mixed coleslaw)
- Allow fish and veg to cool a little before making the rice paper rolls, or the papers will go soft and mushy.
  Use 3 rice paper rounds to make rolls:
- Sliced trout and cooked veg
- Pickled pink sushi ginger
- Greek yoghurt
- Serve with lime wedges and crispy skin on the side.

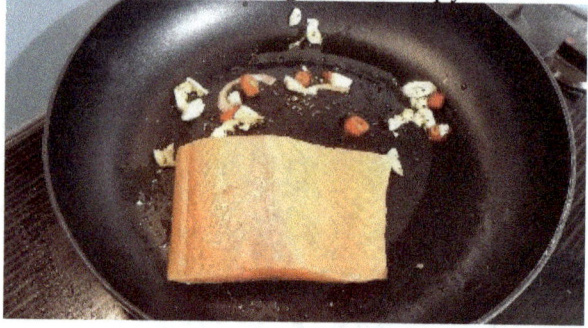

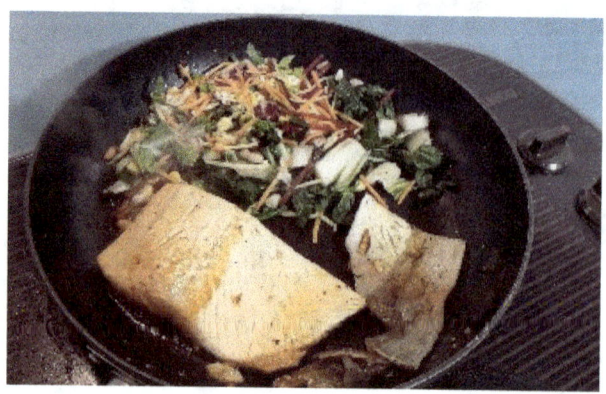

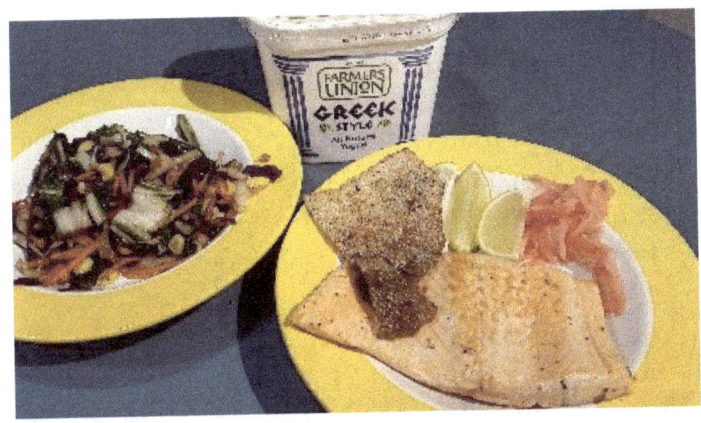
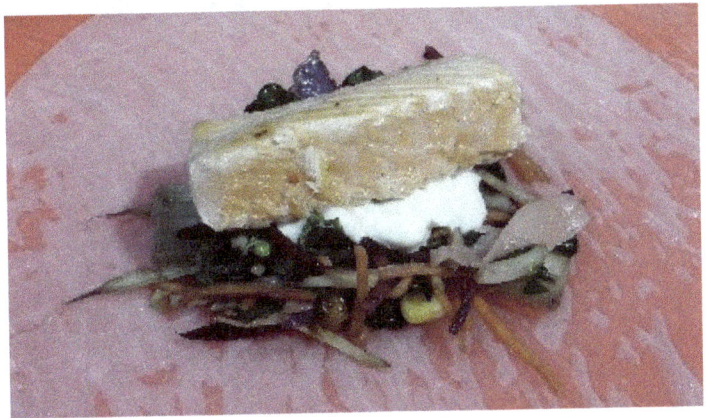
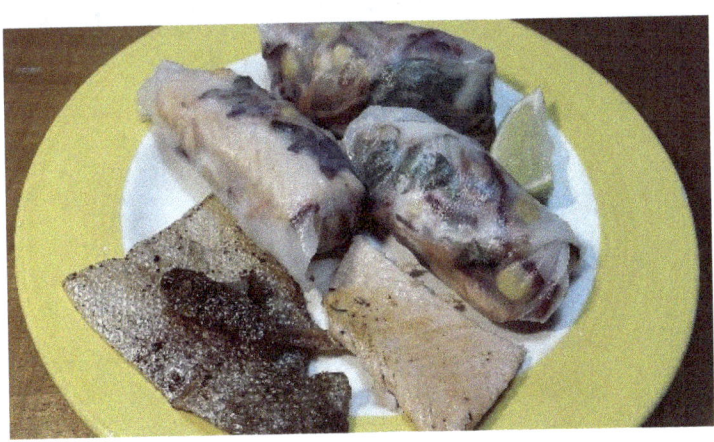

111. Smoked ocean trout rolls

- 3 rice paper rounds
- 100g Ocean Blue Smoked Ocean Trout
- ½ avocado
- Pickled sushi ginger, sliced jalapenos
- Cos lettuce
- Mixed coleslaw/kaleslaw salad (dry)
- Alfalfa sprouts

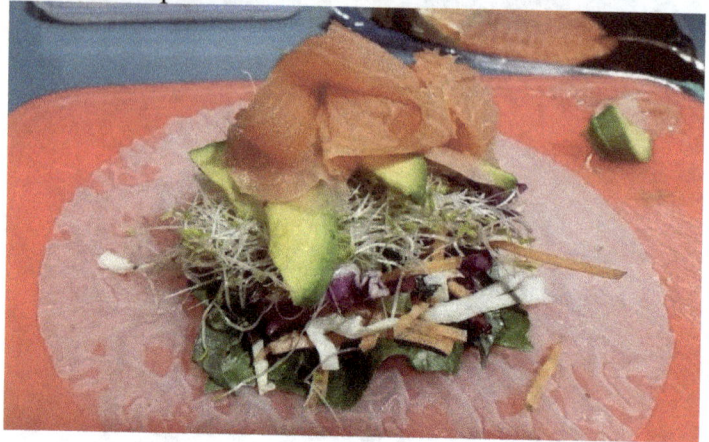

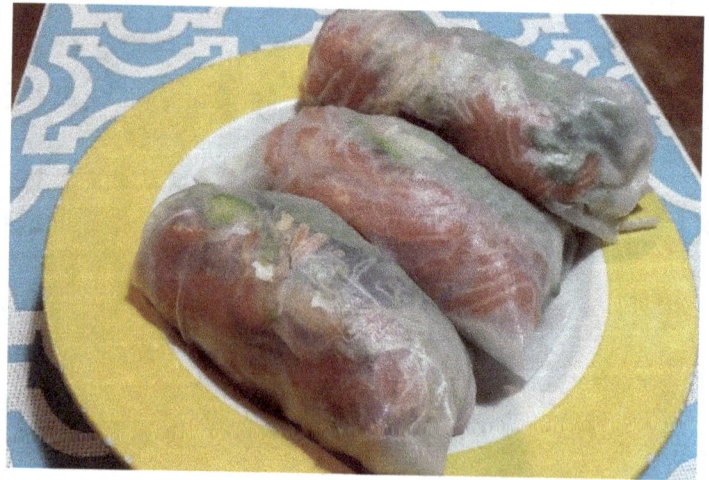

TASMANIAN SALMON

Salmon is a source of protein, omega-3s, vitamins B3, B12 and D, and phosphorus, but much higher in calories than tuna. A fresh fillet of farmed Tasmanian salmon contains more calories than any other fish, so make it a small serve and not too often, if you want to lose weight. But when you do have it, make sure you enjoy it. Buy a piece with the skin on, and cook the skin until it's crispy.

A salmon fillet should be medium-rare, with the centre warm but still pink. If cooking tail fillets, don't overcook the thinner parts. Remove those bits once they're cooked, or prop them up with some vegetables to lift it off the direct heat of the pan.

If making rice paper rolls, allow the cooked fish to cool a little before doing so. A warm filling will make the rice papers go soft too quickly, making them difficult to assemble.

112. Crispy skin salmon, tartare sauce, rolls

- To a hot pan, add olive oil, salt, cracked pepper
- Add fresh fillet of Tasmanian salmon (skin-side down).
- Follow instructions at front of this book, for HOW TO COOK CRISPY SKIN FISH. Season with salt, pepper.
- Allow fish to cool a little before making the rice paper rolls. Slice fish into gougons.

Use 3 rice paper rounds to make rolls:
- Mixed coleslaw and Mizuna salad (with dressing)
- Sliced salmon (warm)
- Pickled pink sushi ginger, jalapenos
- Tartare sauce, chopped dill

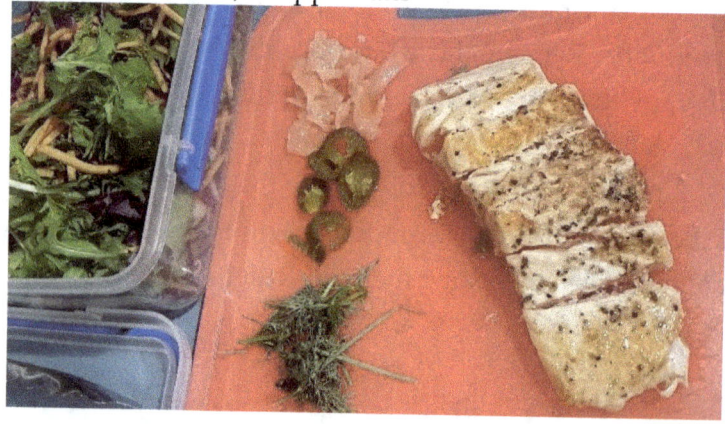

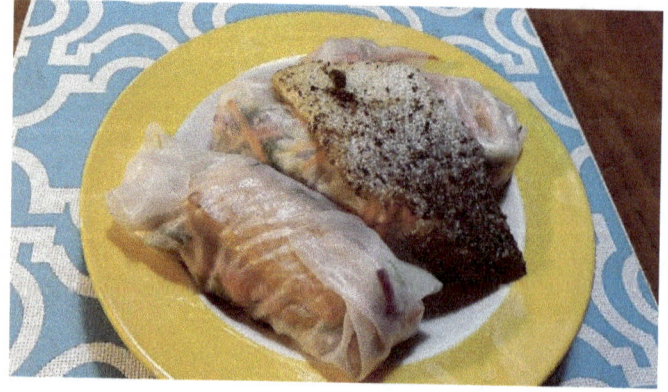

113. Pan-fried salmon cutlet, vegetables

- Pan-fry fresh salmon cutlet in hot pan with olive oil, garlic
- Add vegetables (silverbeet, broccoli, mixed coleslaw veges)
- Squeeze lime juice
- Cook fish on both sides until medium rare, still pink in the middle. Season with salt, cracked pepper.
- Transfer everything to a plate, with lime wedge.

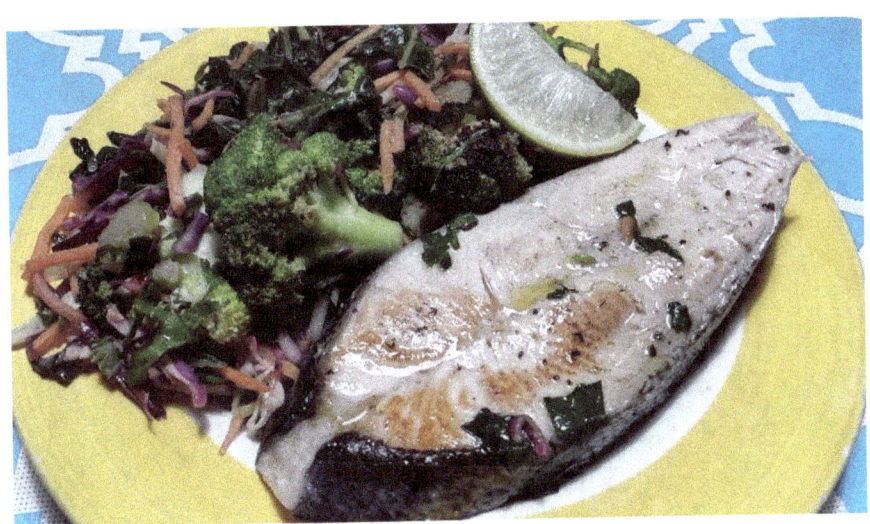

114. Smoked salmon pepper rolls

- 3 rice paper rounds
- 100g Ocean Blue Smoked Salmon Cracked Pepper
- ¼ avocado
- Sliced jalapenos or pickled chili
- Pickled sushi ginger
- Kaleslaw salad mix (dry)

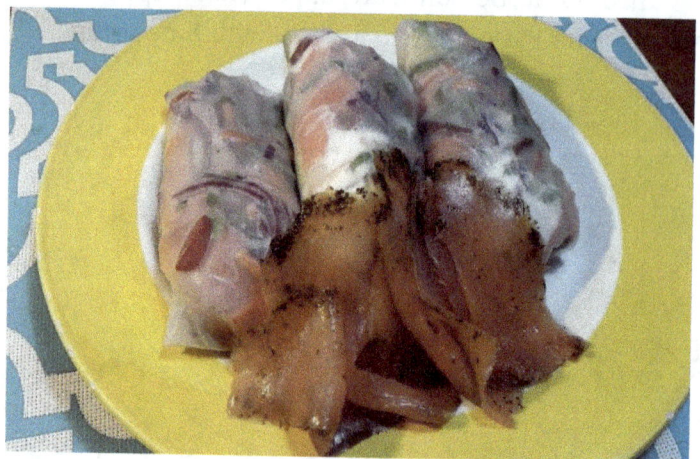

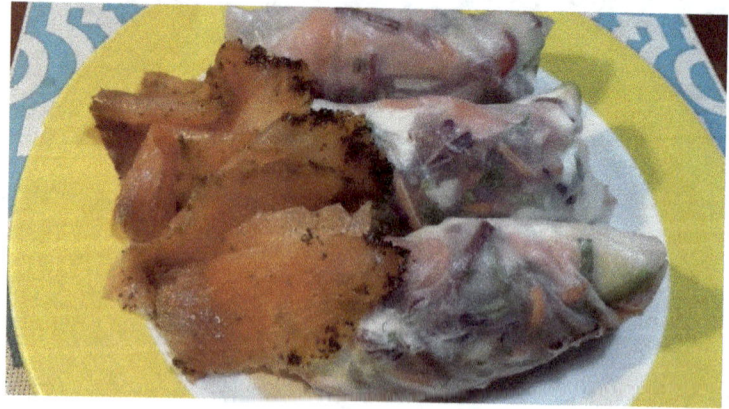

About the author

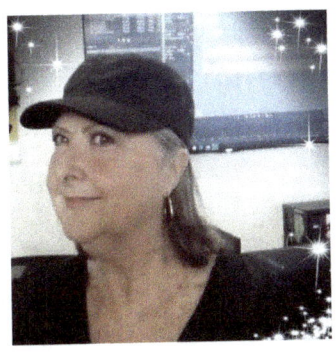

Kathryn M. James

MASR(Health), BScBiomedical(Hons), GDipA(Coun), GDipFDRP

Kathryn M. James is an award-winning Australian author. Her previous book, **THE HUNGER HERO DIET©: How to Lose Weight and Break the Depression Cycle – Without Exercise, Drugs or Surgery**, was the culmination of 10 years of multi-disciplinary studies in the health sciences, combined with the personal experience of depression-related obesity.

This latest work is a companion series of FAST and EASY RECIPES, providing additional resources for anyone who wants to eat better, feel better, and lose weight.

In recent years, Kathryn has achieved academically across five biomedical and behavioural science degrees, worked five years as a Telehealth Counsellor and Psychotherapist helping remote health workers, and she has written numerous magazine articles on food and nutrition. She is now a full-time writer.

Website: https://KMJamesWriter.com/
Email: KMJamesWriter@outlook.com

Titles in the HUNGER HERO series

THE HUNGER HERO DIET: How to Lose Weight and Break the Depression Cycle – Without Exercise, Drugs or Surgery

ISBN	978-0-6455255-0-2	ebook
ISBN	978-0-6455255-1-9	paperback print book
ISBN	978-0-6455255-2-6	hardcover print book

The HUNGER HERO DIET – Fast and Easy Recipe Series #1: Cooking with FISH

ISBN	978-0-6455255-5-7	ebook
ISBN	978-0-6455255-3-3	paperback print book

The HUNGER HERO DIET – Fast and Easy Recipe Series #2: PRAWNS and OTHER SEAFOOD

ISBN	978-0-6455255-6-4	ebook
ISBN	978-0-6455255-4-0	paperback print book

The HUNGER HERO DIET – Fast and Easy Recipe Series #3: Tinned FISH Vietnamese-style

ISBN	978-0-6455255-7-1	ebook